INNOVATIONS IN HEALTH LITERACY RESEARCH

WORKSHOP SUMMARY

Cori Vancheri, *Rapporteur*

Roundtable on Health Literacy
Board on Population Health and Public Health Practice

INSTITUTE OF MEDICINE
OF THE NATIONAL ACADEMIES

THE NATIONAL ACADEMIES PRESS
Washington, D.C.
www.nap.edu

THE NATIONAL ACADEMIES PRESS 500 Fifth Street, N.W. Washington, DC 20001

NOTICE: The project that is the subject of this report was approved by the Governing Board of the National Research Council, whose members are drawn from the councils of the National Academy of Sciences, the National Academy of Engineering, and the Institute of Medicine.

This study was supported by contracts between the National Academy of Sciences and the Agency for Healthcare Research and Quality (HHSP233200900537P), GlaxoSmithKline, Johnson & Johnson, and the Missouri Foundation for Health (09-0290-HL-09). Any opinions, findings, conclusions, or recommendations expressed in this publication are those of the author(s) and do not necessarily reflect the view of the organizations or agencies that provided support for this project.

International Standard Book Number-13: 978-0-309-16185-5
International Standard Book Number-10: 0-309-16185-1

Additional copies of this report are available from the National Academies Press, 500 Fifth Street, N.W., Lockbox 285, Washington, DC 20055; (800) 624-6242 or (202) 334-3313 (in the Washington metropolitan area); Internet, http://www.nap.edu.

For more information about the Institute of Medicine, visit the IOM home page at: **www.iom.edu.**

Printed in the United States of America

The serpent has been a symbol of long life, healing, and knowledge among almost all cultures and religions since the beginning of recorded history. The serpent adopted as a logotype by the Institute of Medicine is a relief carving from ancient Greece, now held by the Staatliche Museen in Berlin.

Suggested citation: IOM (Institute of Medicine). 2011. *Innovations in Health Literacy Research: Workshop Summary.* Washington, DC: The National Academies Press.

"Knowing is not enough; we must apply.
Willing is not enough; we must do."

—Goethe

INSTITUTE OF MEDICINE

OF THE NATIONAL ACADEMIES

Advising the Nation. Improving Health.

THE NATIONAL ACADEMIES

Advisers to the Nation on Science, Engineering, and Medicine

The **National Academy of Sciences** is a private, nonprofit, self-perpetuating society of distinguished scholars engaged in scientific and engineering research, dedicated to the furtherance of science and technology and to their use for the general welfare. Upon the authority of the charter granted to it by the Congress in 1863, the Academy has a mandate that requires it to advise the federal government on scientific and technical matters. Dr. Ralph J. Cicerone is president of the National Academy of Sciences.

The **National Academy of Engineering** was established in 1964, under the charter of the National Academy of Sciences, as a parallel organization of outstanding engineers. It is autonomous in its administration and in the selection of its members, sharing with the National Academy of Sciences the responsibility for advising the federal government. The National Academy of Engineering also sponsors engineering programs aimed at meeting national needs, encourages education and research, and recognizes the superior achievements of engineers. Dr. Charles M. Vest is president of the National Academy of Engineering.

The **Institute of Medicine** was established in 1970 by the National Academy of Sciences to secure the services of eminent members of appropriate professions in the examination of policy matters pertaining to the health of the public. The Institute acts under the responsibility given to the National Academy of Sciences by its congressional charter to be an adviser to the federal government and, upon its own initiative, to identify issues of medical care, research, and education. Dr. Harvey V. Fineberg is president of the Institute of Medicine.

The **National Research Council** was organized by the National Academy of Sciences in 1916 to associate the broad community of science and technology with the Academy's purposes of furthering knowledge and advising the federal government. Functioning in accordance with general policies determined by the Academy, the Council has become the principal operating agency of both the National Academy of Sciences and the National Academy of Engineering in providing services to the government, the public, and the scientific and engineering communities. The Council is administered jointly by both Academies and the Institute of Medicine. Dr. Ralph J. Cicerone and Dr. Charles M. Vest are chair and vice chair, respectively, of the National Research Council.

www.national-academies.org

PLANNING COMMITTEE ON INNOVATIONS IN HEALTH LITERACY RESEARCH*

SHARON E. BARRETT, Health Literacy Staff Consultant, Association of Clinicians for the Underserved

CINDY BRACH, Senior Health Policy Researcher, Agency for Healthcare Research and Quality, U.S. Department of Health and Human Services

JULIE A. GAZMARARIAN, Associate Professor, Emory University Rollins School of Public Health

JEAN KRAUSE, Executive Vice President and CEO, American College of Physicians Foundation

MICHAEL PAASCHE-ORLOW, Associate Professor of Medicine, Boston University School of Medicine

---

* IOM planning committees are solely responsible for organizing the workshop, identifying topics, and choosing speakers. The responsibility for the published workshop summary rests with the workshop rapporteur and the institution.

ROUNDTABLE ON HEALTH LITERACY*

GEORGE ISHAM *(Chair)*, Medical Director and Chief Health Officer, HealthPartners
SHARON E. BARRETT, Health Literacy Staff Consultant, Association of Clinicians for the Underserved
CINDY BRACH, Senior Health Policy Researcher, Center for Delivery, Organization, and Markets, Agency for Healthcare Research and Quality
CAROLYN COCOTAS, Senior Vice President, Quality and Corporate Compliance, F.E.G.S. Health and Human Services System
ARTHUR CULBERT, President and CEO, Health Literacy Missouri
MICHAEL L. DAVIS, Senior Vice President, Human Resources, General Mills, Inc.
BENARD P. DREYER, Professor of Pediatrics, New York University School of Medicine, and Chair, American Academy of Pediatrics Health Literacy Program Advisory Committee
DEBBIE FRITZ, Director, Policy and Standards, Health Management Innovations Division, GlaxoSmithKline
MELODY GOLLER, Health Education Manager, Scientific Activities Division, American Academy of Family Physicians Foundation
MARTHA GRAGG, Vice President of Program, Missouri Foundation for Health
LINDA HARRIS, Team Leader, Health Communication and eHealth Team, Office of Disease Prevention and Health Promotion, U.S. Department of Health and Human Services
BETSY L. HUMPHREYS, Deputy Director, National Library of Medicine, National Institutes of Health
TERRIS KING, Deputy Director, Office of Clinical Standards and Quality, Centers for Medicare & Medicaid Services
JEAN KRAUSE, Executive Vice President and CEO, American College of Physicians Foundation
MARGARET LOVELAND, Global Medical Affairs, Merck & Co., Inc.
RUTH PARKER, Professor of Medicine, Emory University School of Medicine
YOLANDA PARTIDA, Director, National Program Office, Hablamos Juntos, University of California, San Francisco, Fresno Center for Medical Education & Research
CLARENCE PEARSON, Consultant

---

* IOM forums and roundtables do not issue, review, or approve individual documents. The responsibility for the published workshop summary rests with the workshop rapporteur and the institution.

SCOTT C. RATZAN, Vice President, Global Health, Johnson & Johnson
WILL ROSS, Associate Dean for Diversity, Associate Professor of Medicine, Washington University School of Medicine
WILLIAM SMITH, Senior Scientist and Director, Academy for Educational Development
PATRICK WAYTE, Vice President, Marketing and Health Education, American Heart Association
AMY WILSON-STRONKS, Project Director, Division of Standards and Survey Methods, and Principal Investigator, Hospitals, Language, and Culture Study, The Joint Commission
WINSTON F. WONG, Medical Director, Community Benefit, Disparities Improvement and Quality Initiatives, Kaiser Permanente

Study Staff

LYLA M. HERNANDEZ, Senior Program Officer
SUZANNE LANDI, Research Assistant
ROSE MARIE MARTINEZ, Director, Board on Population Health and Public Health Practice

Reviewers

This report has been reviewed in draft form by individuals chosen for their diverse perspectives and technical expertise, in accordance with procedures approved by the National Research Council's Report Review Committee. The purpose of this independent review is to provide candid and critical comments that will assist the institution in making its published report as sound as possible and to ensure that the report meets institutional standards for objectivity, evidence, and responsiveness to the study charge. The review comments and draft manuscript remain confidential to protect the integrity of the process. We wish to thank the following individuals for their review of this report:

Leonard Epstein, Health Resources and Services Administration
Elizabeth Hahn, Northwestern University Feinberg School of Medicine
Alice Horowitz, University of Maryland School of Public Health
Sandra Smith, University of Washington Center for Health Education and Research in Seattle

Although the reviewers listed above have provided many constructive comments and suggestions, they did not endorse the final draft of the report before its release. The review of this report was overseen by **Hugh Tilson**, University of North Carolina School of Public Health. Appointed by the Institute of Medicine, he was responsible for making certain that an independent examination of this report was carried out in accordance with institutional procedures and that all review comments were carefully considered. Responsibility for the final content of this report rests entirely with the rapporteur and the institution.

Acknowledgments

The support of the sponsors of the Institute of Medicine Roundtable on Health Literacy made it possible to plan and conduct the workshop on innovations in health literacy research which this report summarizes. Sponsorship for the Roundtable comes from the Agency for Healthcare Research and Quality, GlaxoSmithKline, Johnson & Johnson, and the Missouri Foundation for Health.

The Roundtable wishes to express its appreciation to Michael Paasche-Orlow for preparation and presentation of a paper summarizing the Health Literacy Annual Research Conference. The Roundtable is also grateful to Lisa Cooper and Dean Schillenger for their presentations on the role of health literacy in health disparities research; to Joshua Seidman and Michael Wolf for their presentations on health literacy in health information technology; and to David Baker and Debra Roter for their presentations on building the field of health literacy research. Thanks also go to Cynthia Baur for presentation of the HHS National Action Plan to Improve Health Literacy; to Carolyn Clancy and Raynard Kingdon for their presentations on the importance of the National Action Plan; and to Terry Davis and Rima Rudd for their presentations on the role of health literacy research in the National Action Plan.

The Roundtable would also like to thank the members of the workshop planning committee for their efforts in developing an excellent workshop agenda. Members of the planning committee were Sharon Barrett, Cindy Brach, Julie Gazmararian, Jean Krause, and Michael Paasche-Orlow.

Contents

TABLE

FIGURES

1

Introduction

The past two decades of research in health literacy have done much to raise awareness about the problems associated with low health literacy. Health literacy is defined as "the degree to which individuals have the capacity to obtain, process, and understand basic health information and services needed to make appropriate health decisions (Ratzan and Parker, 2000). Nearly 9 out of 10 adults have difficulty using everyday health information that is available in health care facilities, retail outlets, media, and communities (ODPHP, 2010). The impact of low health literacy disproportionately affects lower socioeconomic and minority groups (Kutner et al, 2006). With knowledge of the effect of low health literacy, what does research say can be done to improve health literacy? Do interventions exist—aimed at either the consumer and patient or the healthcare system—that have been tested and shown to be effective? What research is needed to change the state of health literacy in the United States?

The Institute of Medicine Roundtable on Health Literacy focuses on building partnerships to move the field of health literacy forward by translating research findings into practical strategies for implementation. The roundtable serves to educate the public, press, and policy makers regarding issues of health literacy. The roundtable sponsors workshops for members and the public to discuss approaches to resolve key challenges in the field. A planning group designed a workshop to explore areas for research in health literacy, including the relationship of health literacy to health disparities and information technology applications. The role of the workshop planning committee was limited to planning the workshop. Unlike a consensus committee report, a workshop summary may not contain conclusions and recommendations. Therefore, this summary has been prepared by the workshop rapporteur as a factual summary of what occurred at the workshop.

The workshop was moderated by George Isham. It began with a presentation about the first annual Health Literacy Annual Research Conference (HARC), held in October 2009. Discussion focused on two of the recurring themes of the HARC meeting: the integration of research on health literacy and health disparities; and the role of information technology and health literacy research. For the workshop summarized in this report, a panel was convened to address each of the two themes described above. The third workshop panel focused on professional development in health literacy research. In the fourth panel, leaders of three government agencies offered the first public presentation of the new National Action Plan to Improve Health Literacy. The final workshop panel addressed the role of health literacy research in the National Action Plan. The workshop ended with a discussion of lessons learned from the workshop.

2

Report on the First Annual Research on Health Literacy Conference

MICHAEL PAASCHE-ORLOW, MD, MA, MPH

Boston University School of Medicine

The problem of low health literacy has been acknowledged, Paasche-Orlow said. Now researchers are trying to figure out how to do something about it. A great deal of research is needed because, while there has been an increase in publications on health literacy, the majority of studies have been observational, with very few clinical trials.

The Health Literacy Annual Research Conference (HARC) was created as an interdisciplinary meeting for investigators who are dedicated to health literacy research with two aims: to advance the science of health literacy research and to serve as an engine to promote professional development in the field. The first meeting, held in October 2009, had two themes: the role of health literacy research in the elimination of health disparities, and health literacy and health information technology. After keynote addresses on the role of health literacy in patient education[1] and on the role of health literacy in health disparities,[2] four panels of invited speakers discussed measurement; health literacy and verbal interactions; health information technology (HIT) interventions; and organizational assessment and change. Current gaps in the research were examined by invited speakers and in breakout sessions relating to public health

[1] By David Baker, Northwestern University.

[2] By Anne Beal, Aetna Foundation.

approaches to health literacy, health disparities and health literacy, and health IT. All of the presentation slides are available on the conference website.[3] A special issue of the *Journal of Health Communication*, guest edited by Paasche-Orlow, Lauren McCormack, and Elizabeth Wilson, reported on the HARC meeting and was published in September 2010, with free full text access online for 6 months.[4] HARC II took place October 18-20, 2010, during the preparation of this report.

Limited health literacy has been linked to worse health outcomes for a range of medical conditions, Paasche-Orlow said. In addition, limited health literacy is more prevalent in specific racial and ethnic minorities. Although these findings have been widely acknowledged, little systematic research has been conducted to elucidate the role of health literacy in the creation of health disparities or to evaluate the possibility that interventions relating to health literacy may help eliminate health disparities.

In thinking about underlying contributions to health disparities, one perspective is that unneeded complexity in public health and health care systems transforms underlying educational disparities in our society into health disparities. Therefore, health literacy can be a roadmap to developing interventions to address health disparities. To differentiate the pathways through which people experience worse outcomes, both health disparities and health literacy need to be measured.

In a study of 204 patients with HIV, an initial analysis did not include literacy (Osborn et al., 2007). Results appeared to show that African American patients were much more likely to not adhere to their HIV medication regimen than whites. But when literacy was controlled for, the race effect diminished. The literacy variable was the only significant independent predictor of nonadherence. Those two very different results would lead to different types of interventions.

In a second study, patients were asked their preference regarding end-of-life care if they developed advanced dementia (Volandes et al., 2008). In an analysis that did not consider health literacy, African-American subjects appeared to be much more likely to want more aggressive care at the end of life. A handful of other studies support this conclusion. But the studies typically do not control for socioeconomic factors, and certainly not literacy. When controlling for health literacy in the study by Volandes and colleagues (2008), the race finding evaporated, and health literacy was found to be the dominant predictor of wanting more aggressive care at the end of life. Finally, when subjects were shown an educational video, differences by race as well as health literacy dropped. The preference for

[3] See www.bumc.bu.edu/healthliteracyconference/2009-conference/.

[4] See http://www.gwu.edu/~cih/journal/.

aggressive care was not a true underlying cultural preference, but rather a misunderstanding and lack of communication about end-of-life care.

In the studies discussed above, as stated previously, analyses that control for health literacy and those that do not, yield vastly different responses. If the issue is one of cultural differences, clinicians are asked to respect and protect that preference. But if the issue is a literacy issue different interventions are needed, interventions that address the issue of poor health literacy.

The second theme of the HARC conference was health literacy and health information technology. Much of the motivation to work in health literacy revolves around the desire to address the needs of vulnerable populations. How will patients with limited literacy skills be able to access technologies? And if they obtain access, will they be able to use the technologies? The open marketplace may not serve the patients with limited literacy. What needs to be done, Paasche-Orlow said, is to make sure that as the health IT movement gains momentum, it does not exacerbate disparities. It is probable that advances in health IT will, in the short term increase disparities, he said. But if work is done now, perhaps that can be overcome.

Across two different intervention studies, to be published in the special issue of the *Journal of Health Communication*, researchers found that people with limited literacy are able use health IT systems. In these studies, an interface that talked to users who responded by touching the screen was used, demonstrating that it is possible to build an interface that people can and will use.

Health literacy research takes a long time, both to obtain funding and to implement. But the research itself is a form of advocacy. By examining the effect of health literacy on different aspects of health care and health outcomes, researchers can reveal interventions that might work to eliminate or reduce problems, Paasche-Orlow concluded.

3

The Role of Health Literacy in Health Disparities Research

HEALTH LITERACY AND HEALTH DISPARITIES: OPPORTUNITIES FOR TRANS-DISCIPLINARY COLLABORATION

Lisa Cooper, M.D., M.P.H.
Johns Hopkins Bloomberg School of Public Health

Health literacy is defined as the capacity to obtain, process, and understand basic health information and services to make appropriate decisions about health (IOM, 2004). Health disparities have been defined by the federal government as differences in health that occur by particular categories: gender, race or ethnicity, income and education, disability, living in a rural locality, or sexual orientation (HHS, 2006). Literacy is not mentioned, although education may have some correlation with health literacy.

In conceptual models of health literacy, cultural and other social factors are mentioned as influencing health literacy (Figure 3-1), but how those factors exert influence is not explicitly described.

The models do show, however, that health disparities are multifactorial, resulting from the interaction of a variety of factors: socioeconomic and environmental (where people live, neighborhood conditions), psychosocial factors (stress, exposure to discrimination), health behaviors, access to care, and quality of care.

Health literacy has not been an explicit issue in disparities research until recently. Where does health literacy fit within a disparities framework? Is it a health risk behavior, as are poor dietary habits or exercise,

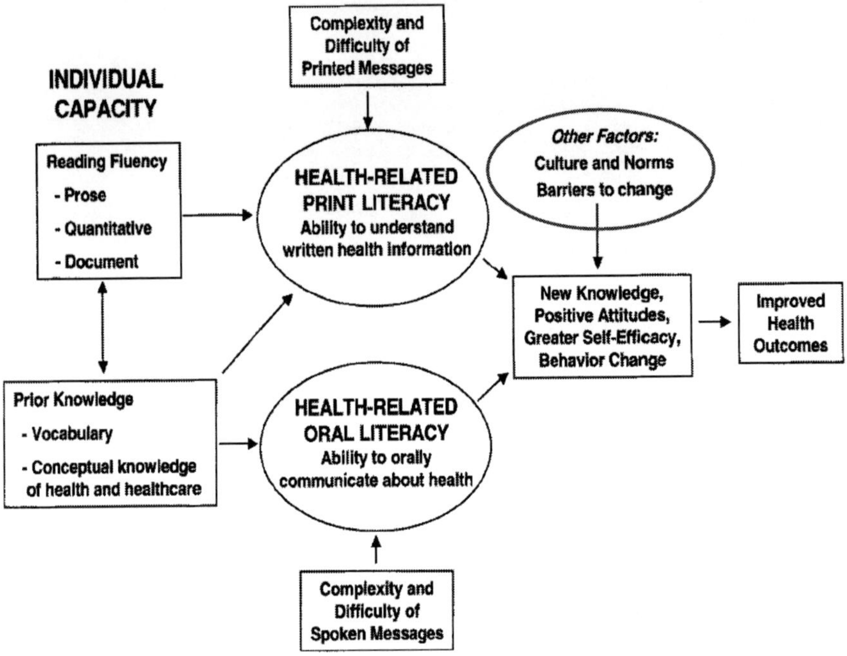

FIGURE 3-1 Conceptual model of health literacy.
SOURCE: Baker (2006).

or smoking or use of alcohol or drugs? Is it a psychosocial factor? Is it a biological factor?

Some models of health disparities have been modified to examine health literacy and language as barriers to access to health care (Figure 3-2).

In a brief PubMed search using the terms *health literacy* and *health disparities*, Cooper said she identified 161 articles; 26 of them were reviews. Some studies were descriptive, comparing health literacy prevalence across disparity conditions. Others showed that disparities in health literacy between disparity populations and majority populations contributed to differences in access and quality of care. Fewer studies examined health literacy as a mediator of disparities in health outcomes. Far fewer studies looked at interventions being tested with low-literacy patients who also belonged to disparity populations to see if these interventions would reduce disparities.

It is interesting to note, Cooper said, that health disparities research has evolved in a manner similar to health literacy research. They both began by describing problems in different populations, then moved into

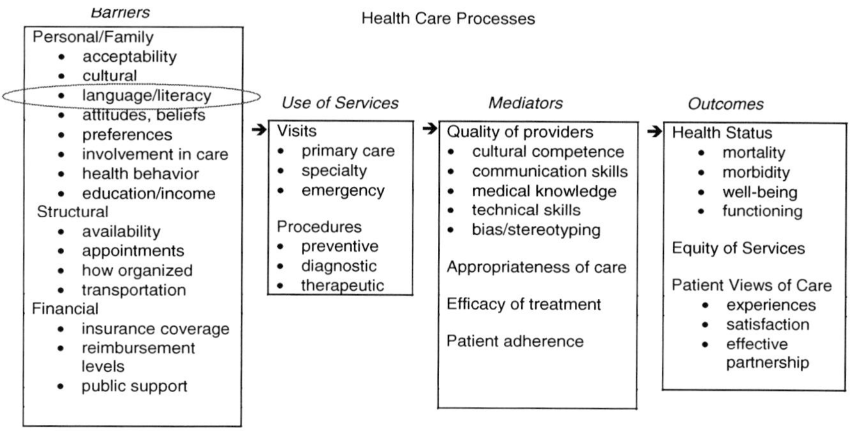

FIGURE 3-2 Understanding disparities in access to and quality of health care.
SOURCE: Cooper et al., 2002.

research aimed at understanding mechanisms of the problems, and now research is moving toward designing interventions and evaluating outcomes. Health disparities and health literacy research also share some common themes and challenges. In both areas there is a documented burden and impact of being in those risk categories. Both affect access, healthcare quality, and outcomes—across numerous conditions and for various populations. In pediatric populations, if there is low literacy in the parents, the children experience disparities.

Also, there is a need for better measurement of key constructs. In health disparities research, for example, better measures are needed for determining specific ethnic groups and language ability. The same is true for health literacy measures, Cooper said. Furthermore, researchers need to better understand mechanisms that explain how belonging in the risk category of health literacy or of health disparities influences outcomes. People in each category experience bias or discrimination with regard to health care. And problems with health disparities as well as health literacy require effective interventions that work across diverse groups. There are many things that the two fields could do together.

Researchers in both fields have tried common intervention strategies (Chin et al., 2007; Sudore and Schillinger, 2009). Some focused on the clinician–patient relationship, such as targeting communications to overcome language or cultural barriers, and other strategies are systems based. For example, patients receive health education information, or are put in self-management support groups. Sometimes, the clinical environment is changed to suit cultural or linguistic needs. Common intervention strategies at the clinician–patient level include patient-centered or clear communication techniques and overcoming cultural or language barriers. At the system patient level, strategies are clear health education materials and audiovisual aids, self-management support programs, and culturally and linguistically tailored clinical environments. Community interventions include social service referrals, use of lay health educators, and mass media (Chin et al., 2007; Sudore and Schillinger, 2009).

There are differences between the two areas as well (Table 3-1). For example, low health literacy is potentially modifiable and a person's literacy status is not readily apparent. Being part of a disparity category such as being of a certain race or age, however, is not subject to change and is mostly visible. There are some challenges that result from these differences between the two areas.

Health literacy research and health disparities research are interdisciplinary in nature, involving many of the same disciplines. How can these two areas of research be brought together? According to Robertson and colleagues (2003) there are several questions to consider in determining if there is a need for interdisciplinary collaboration. Which fields have been included or excluded thus far? How thoroughly should the researchers exploit the opportunity for interdisciplinary collaboration? For instance, is there a need to devise a new common vocabulary and new methods?

How important are institutions in facilitating or thwarting the process? How key is the integration of disciplinary perspectives in fashioning a more powerful explanation of the phenomenon in question? There are many disciplines that have potential contributions to make to health literacy and health disparities research, including experts from behavioral science, sociology, social work, speech and language, organizational behavior, social psychology, health services research, epidemiology, cultural anthropology, bioethics, biostatistics, economics, cognitive psychology, neuropsychology, education and learning, psychometrics, health

TABLE 3.1 Contrasting Themes

Health Literacy	Health Disparities
Low health literacy is potentially modifiable	Population assignment usually not modifiable
Literacy status not readily apparent	Disparity category (e.g., race, gender, age) mostly visible
Internally defined, individually experienced	Externally defined, socially driven and experienced

professionals and policy experts. How can they be encouraged to work together? What are the structural and cognitive barriers? Structural barriers include time, space, funding, and infrastructure issues (Richter and Paretti, 2008). Cognitive barriers include lack of awareness, relatedness, and perspective. For example, health literacy researchers may be focused on that particular area because of their sensitivities to it, but they may not have the sense of how connected it could be to a disparity problem. These barriers need to be overcome.

There are ways to address the structural barriers, such as creating convenient meeting times, holding special sessions at annual meetings of professional societies that are attended by both disciplines, creating informal networks so that work groups and social communal gatherings can occur in neutral, permanent space. A special journal or special issues devoted to health literacy and disparities research is another option as is making use of virtual collaboration options such as chat rooms, mail lists, and shared networks. Organizing funding priorities by cutting across themes is vital, Cooper said.

To enhance awareness of each field of research for the other, bring people together and encourage conversation. Ask each discipline to talk about what it does, its measurement and study design strategies, and the challenges and constraints it faces. Look for commonalities. To enhance relatedness and perspective, bring people together to define the problems and criteria together. Have them work together to develop measurement instruments to enhance their validity. Foster cross-disciplinary pairing, for example, use co-PIs (co-principal investigators) on projects who are from different disciplines. One example is the National Institutes of Health (NIH) Common Fund Program[1] which supports a series of cross-cutting, trans-NIH research programs, including new programs in the science of behavior change and global health. It creates research consortia, establishes interdisciplinary training initiatives, promotes interdisciplinary technology methods, and has a multiple PI policy. Perhaps health literacy and health disparities could be the next topic for the NIH Common Fund program.

A roadmap for collaboration between health disparities and health literacy researchers would include several stages. First, it is important to determine which issues or questions would benefit from having researchers from the two disciplines come together. Pertinent questions include the following: Are tests of health literacy valid across populations? Is literacy causally related to health disparities or a marker for some other risk factor not yet identified? Which particular aspects of health literacy are most relevant for different disparity populations? In which settings

[1] See http://nihroadmap.nih.gov/.

or contexts do health literacy and other disparity conditions interact to worsen health? What are the mechanisms by which literacy contributes to disparities? Are links to outcomes present in nationally representative samples?

It will be important to obtain agreement from both fields of research that the interdisciplinary approach is necessary to adequately address research questions. Because the conceptual models for health disparities and health literacy do not bring the two fields together in a comprehensive way, it is important to anticipate potential communication issues among the participants from disparate disciplines and promote frequent communication (electronic and face-to-face meetings) to enhance opportunities for dialogue and information exchange. Such communication will facilitate the combining of empirical and theoretical methodologies to test new models.

Other steps needed to promote collaboration are: include a broad range of disciplines through proactive selection as well as self-selection; create a framework to guide the unique interdisciplinary research effort, each participant's contribution, and training initiatives; and add appropriate literacy-related measurement to epidemiological studies and nationally representative samples.

In summary, Cooper said, health literacy and health disparities research have evolved in a similar manner. The two disciplines share themes, challenges, and intervention strategies. However, some differences exist in the extent to which belonging to a literacy category or disparity category is modifiable, how it is viewed by others, and how it is experienced by the individual. Finally, interdisciplinary collaboration will require overcoming the structural and cognitive barriers discussed.

WILL IMPROVING HEALTH LITERACY REDUCE HEALTH DISPARITIES FOR VULNERABLE POPULATIONS?

Dean Schillinger, M.D.
University of California, San Francisco
San Francisco General Hospital

Asking whether improving health literacy will reduce health disparities for vulnerable populations is a challenging question. To answer this we must first determine if we can improve health literacy in vulnerable populations. Second, if we do improve health literacy, will *disparity populations* or vulnerable populations disproportionately benefit? Schillinger said that he intended to address four questions in his presentation:

- Does health literacy explain health disparities by race and education?
- What are hypothesized mechanisms by which better health literacy can improve health for vulnerable populations?
- What evidence exists that health literacy interventions improve health for vulnerable populations?
- What is the need for a "vulnerable populations approach" to improving health literacy?

Vulnerable populations have been described as subgroups that, because of shared social characteristics, are at higher risk of risks. This implies that their vulnerability is socially determined by the structural nature of a society, and that vulnerable populations, by virtue of being vulnerable, are much more likely to be at high risk of being exposed to risk of illness. Vulnerable populations are exposed to contextual conditions that distinguish them from the rest of the population.

In public health practice in the United States, vulnerable groups are generally considered to be (a) certain race and ethnic minorities, (b) low income, (c) those with a high school diploma or less, and (d) immigrants and those with limited English proficiency. Only (a) and (c) on this list have been studied with respect to the question of whether health literacy explains some of the relationships between social characteristics and health outcomes.

Six positive cross-sectional studies have explored health literacy's impact on socioeconomic disparities and health outcomes. Bennett and colleagues (2009) studied nearly 3,000 adults over age 65 who participated in the National Assessment of Adult of Literacy (NAAL) and found that health literacy mediated the relationship between educational attainment and self-rated health, receipt of flu vaccines, receipt of mammograms, and dental care. Howard and colleagues (2006) studied more than 3,000 seniors from the Prudential Study and found that health literacy explained the relationship between education and physical and mental health scores, but not preventive care use, such as flu vaccine, mammograms, and dental care. Yin and colleagues (2009) studied parents who participated in NAAL and found that health literacy mediated the relationship between educational attainment and health-literacy-related tasks regarding child health, dosing medications, and pediatrician appointments.

Sentell and Halpin (2006) studied 24,000 participants in National Adult Literacy Survey performed in the 1990s and found that literacy mediated the relationship between education and the presence of chronic illness and a health condition that limited ability to function in society. Sarkar and colleagues (2010) studied more than 14,000 patients with diabetes in the Kaiser Permanente health plan and found that literacy strongly mediated the relationship between educational attainment and patient's use of the electronic patient portal. Finally, Schillinger and colleagues (2006) studied public hospital patients with diabetes and found that health literacy mediated the relationship between education and hemoglobin A1c. In all the studies, mediation was partial; health literacy is not a full explanation of the relationship.

On the question of whether health literacy explains race and ethnic disparities in health outcomes, six cross-sectional studies—some already mentioned, some additional—have looked at the explanatory power of health literacy with respect to black/white differences in health outcomes, and none has looked at other ethnic differences. Bennett and colleagues (2009) found that health literacy mediated the relationship between race and self-rated health and flu vaccine receipt, but not mammography or dental care. In the Prudential study, Howard and colleagues (2006) found that health literacy mediated the relationship between race and mental health but not physical health and not receipt of preventive care.

Sentell and Halpin (2006) found that literacy mediated the relationship between race and long-term illness and a limiting health condition, just as it did with education. Bailey and colleagues (2009) studied 373 parents and found that health literacy mediated the relationship between African Americans and whites, and misunderstandings about liquid medication dosing. Osborn and colleagues (2009), studying patients with diabetes, found that diabetes-related numeracy mediated the relationship between race and hemoglobin A1c. In patients with prostate cancer, Wolf and colleagues (2006) found that health literacy mediated the relationship between race and the level of prostate-specific-antigen (PSA) at the time of presentation with prostate cancer. The only before and after trial (Volandes et al., 2008) found that health literacy mediated the relationship between race and changes in advanced care preferences. After viewing a video, patient preferences, especially among those with low literacy, changed to preferring less aggressive care.

All but one of the large studies are cross-sectional. This raises a number of questions, but the largest question is one of causation. Interpreting these studies requires caution. There are multiple opportunities for confounding. Limited literacy may be a marker for social disadvantage. What happens in early childhood development can codetermine limited literacy and worse health trajectories. Another concern is that health literacy can be mismeasured across race and ethnicity. When we use the REALM (Rapid Estimate of Adult Literacy in Medicine) or other approaches to health literacy measurement in an African American or Latino patient, are we really measuring health literacy? Or are we detecting differences in social strata that are really determining people's health trajectory?

Is the observed mediation taking place at the community level rather than individual level, since health is shaped for vulnerable populations within the important social context where health care is received? Are there health mediators at the neighborhood level that are driving the relationships? Or is there a cyclical relationship, that is, does illness trajectory lead to lower scores on a literacy test that are associated with a worse health trajectory? Finally, is there something happening in the fragmented health care system that leads to suboptimal or discriminatory quality of care and premature death and morbidity?

What Are the Hypothesized Mechanisms by Which Better Health Literacy Can Improve Health for Vulnerable Populations?

There are several hypothesized mechanisms that link health literacy, health disparities, and health outcomes. There is growing evidence that suggests that limited health literacy is associated with a higher incidence of disease burden of illness, especially chronic disease. While it is reasonable to assume that the person with limited literacy who cannot read the label might eat the unhealthy food that then leads to sickness, the association may also be a reflection of a contextual problem, Schillinger said. Those with limited literacy, because of the clustering of risks, are more likely to be living in a neighborhood under circumstances that are associated with high rates of chronic disease.

Occupational risk and exposures are also linked to one's literacy skills and may lead to poorer health. Another mechanism may be that those with limited health literacy have a lower degree of health awareness and are less likely to have early recognition of symptoms. Fang and colleagues (2009) studied patients on warfarin, a medication to prevent stroke. She was able to demonstrate that only 1 in 10 patients reported that the purpose of taking warfarin was to reduce risk of stroke. Among English- and Spanish-speaking participants, inadequate literacy was strongly associated with discordant responses about the nature of stroke, and very few patients could accurately report a symptom of stroke. Being at high risk of stroke but unable to know what a typical sign or symptom is could lead to negative stroke outcomes.

Accessing and navigating complex health and social service systems is clearly a mechanism that may disproportionately affect vulnerable populations, Schillinger said. In California, for example, people have to reapply for Medicare every 3 months, which contributes to higher turnover in health coverage and access to care problems. Additionally, there is a concern and growing body of evidence in the health disparities field that suggest that diffusion and uptake of innovations in health care is a mechanism that contributes to disparities. In health IT, that can be particularly problematic with respect to navigation.

Another possible mechanism relates to adherence. There is some evidence that low health literacy leads to problems with *accuracy* in medication administration and errors (e.g. unintentional nonadherence) as opposed to intentional nonadherence. And clearly, health literacy is a barrier to learning and the performance of self-management behaviors.

It is now recognized that communication in the clinic encounter is often severely impaired. Health professionals are not successfully communicating with patients who have limited health literacy—regarding medication reconciliation, patient history, discussing symptoms and barriers to care in the absence of a physician eliciting it, and patient understanding of explanations and results and whether they ask questions. Finally, the ethical processes that underpin trust and the clinician–patient relationship, such as shared decision making, articulating preferences, and providing informed consent are potential mechanisms linking health literacy, health disparities, and health outcomes.

What Evidence Exists That Health Literacy Interventions Improve Health for Vulnerable Populations?

Turning to the question of whether health literacy intervention reduces disparities, there is much less data. Most studies evaluating health literacy interventions have demonstrated improvements that disproportionately accrue to those with adequate health literacy, or they yield similar improvements across health literacy. Most studies do not report the effects on vulnerable subgroups by, for example, stratifying results by race ethnicity or educational attainment.

A few health literacy interventions have been found to disproportionately affect vulnerable subgroups. Rothman and colleagues (2004) tested a health-literacy-sensitive diabetes management program that disproportionately benefited those with limited health literacy compared with those who had adequate health literacy. DeWalt and colleagues (2006) did the same on congestive heart failure. Paasche-Orlow and colleagues (2005) used a teach-to-goal approach in asthma education, which disproportionately benefited those with limited health literacy versus those with adequate health literacy. An automated diabetes phone system disproportionately engaged and led to behavior change among those with limited literacy and limited English proficiency compared with others (Schillinger et al., 2008). Finally, work by Machtinger and colleagues (2007) found visual medication schedules, when combined with a "teach back" in anticoagulation care, disproportionately benefited those with communication barriers.

Reducing disparities requires taking a socioecological approach, Schillinger said, This approach includes thinking about the context in which people live and receive their healthcare. An important question to consider is, will better *individual* health literacy lead people to make healthier choices, particularly those who are in vulnerable populations? Given the cluster of risks that vulnerable populations face—food insecurity, food access problems, unsafe neighborhoods, and so on—that are determined by social context, it is important to be realistic regarding expectations of what improving health literacy can do.

Another important issue is whether attempts to affect individual health literacy will be hampered by the nature of health systems that disproportionately care for vulnerable populations. Varkey and colleagues (2009) studied primary care practices stratified by the proportion of minority patients served. Practices that served 30 percent or more minority patients were compared to practices with fewer minorities. Tremendous differences were found in organizational structure, workforce satisfaction, comorbidity, complexity of disease, and perceived practice chaos. Work settings significantly affect the health care provided to vulnerable populations.

Context is important. Preliminary evidence suggests these factors can affect the relationship between health literacy and outcomes. In studies of the relationship between health literacy and chronic disease control (e.g., blood pressure, diabetes), whether or not there is a relationship between health literacy and the outcome appears to vary based on the setting. Schillinger's work at a public hospital showed a clear relationship between health literacy and diabetes outcomes, but a similar replication study in a private setting in New England found no relationship (Morris et al, 2006) and a study of literacy and blood pressure control found that the relationship varied by setting (Powers BJ 2008). Contextual factors need further analysis.

What Is the Need for a "Vulnerable Populations Approach" to Improving Health Literacy?

There are three commonly described public health intervention approaches. The first is Lalonde's at-risk approach. This approach targets those with high-risk behaviors for specific conditions (Lalonde, 1974). An example of this is targeting smokers to reduce cardiovascular disease. The second approach is Rose's population approach (Rose, 1992), which focuses on those with the average risk exposure, which is really the entire population. Interventions are designed to shift the curve in order to achieve the greatest public health benefit by improving population health. The third approach has been articulated by Frohlich and Potvin (2008) and is known as the vulnerable populations approach. This approach focuses on fundamental causes, on life course trajectories, and on the concentration of risk in vulnerable subgroups. The Lalonde and Rose approaches may be neutral with respect to reducing disparities, or could exacerbate disparities. For example, electronic health records (EHRs) may be of benefit to the general population but may leave vulnerable populations behind (Sarkar et al., 2010), and therefore exacerbate disparities.

Successful approaches need to combine Rose's population approach with Frohlich's vulnerable population approach. Schillinger said. Improvements in population health must be linked with reductions in disparities. While general populations can be targeted for improvements in health, the targets for special intervention should be vulnerable populations in the context of the settings that care for them and the neighborhoods in which they live. The work has to be multi-sectorial—for example, schools and health care settings—it needs to be participatory, and it needs to address upstream determinants.

In conclusion, Schillinger said, health literacy may be a mediator of social disparities in health outcomes, but many questions remain. More research is needed, taking a socioecological, multilevel, and life course approach. Health literacy interventions have the potential to reduce disparities, but they often do not. If better health literacy is to reduce health disparities, interventions will need to target vulnerable populations where they live and where they receive services.

DISCUSSION

Cindy Brach, Agency for Healthcare Research and Quality, said it makes sense to concentrate resources on the needs of vulnerable populations, but, she asked, what about approaches that appeal to a wide spectrum since they have the potential to benefit everybody? Schillinger responded that he would call for a two-tiered approach, addressing the entire population with focused efforts on vulnerable subgroups for whom the problem is most severe. With just the population approach, one runs the risk of increasing disparities. He pointed to the electronic health records example at Kaiser, where the data show an increase in disparities. His guess is that a participatory approach to developing the EHR was not used. Winston Wong, roundtable member from Kaiser Permanente, said that Kaiser did use user groups in the design of portions of the new EHR system. There is evidence of disproportionate use among different populations. Kaiser is planning a policy roundtable to look more closely at this issue. Schillinger said that, despite the difficulties encountered, what Kaiser is doing is ahead of the curve, a harbinger of the future. Incorporating the health literacy principles into the meaningful use definition of health IT is very important.

Paasche-Orlow noted that in some of the examples, a generalized approach was especially beneficial to groups with the highest need.

With either approach, it is important to measure the effects on the at-risk population. There are those who think that simplifying and standardizing things will benefit all, although it might benefit some more than others.

Cooper noted the commonality of themes between health disparities and health literacy research. Health disparities share the same concern about using universal approaches and standard quality improvements that could improve the situation overall, but may exacerbate disparities. It is important to look for unintended consequences.

Benard Dreyer, roundtable member and pediatrician from New York University School of Medicine, asked if there is evidence that universal interventions are better than targeted interventions for vulnerable populations. If vulnerable populations are at highest risk for poor outcomes due to low literacy, would targeted outcomes be more effective, especially if the interventions needed for low literacy populations may not be acceptable to other populations? The American Academy of Pediatrics (AAP) produced low-literacy patient education materials, which the AAP thinks are not going to be acceptable to higher literacy populations.

Cooper said she is philosophically in agreement on targeting vulnerable groups, but she encounters much resistance. People who manage health services ask why such targeted interventions are necessary as they can be more cost intensive and more labor intensive. Researchers must demonstrate to decision makers that a tailored or targeted approach is more effective than a standard, universal approach. This has not yet been shown. There is also the difficulty of measuring and determining who are the vulnerable, which is not always easy. By making assumptions about who the vulnerable are and targeting them, others who could benefit from the intervention may be missed.

Schillinger said that the typical costs of the public health type of intervention are low and are shared across society, whereas the cost associated with targeted, tailored interventions tend to be greater and focused on fewer people, which is a harder case to make for policy makers. Paasche-Orlow questioned how much tailoring is really necessary. It can be endless, and there will always be other groups that need tailored interventions. The trick with the five interventions that appear to reduce disparities, said Schillinger, is that many are universal precautions, but embedded in them is the fact that those who need more, get more. If it takes three rounds to teach a patient how to use the asthma inhaler, then three rounds it is. It may work to embed that sort of logic, so those who need more in an intervention get more.

Arthur Culbert, roundtable member from Health Literacy Missouri, stated that the challenge in Missouri is whether to address everyone or target certain groups. The factors mentioned today—cost, disparities, and health literacy issues—are real. It is worth trying a variety of scenarios to see what works, he said.

Wong asked if the HARC conference planners intend to discuss the system changes that will be introduced given health care reforms. For example, individuals will have to make choices regarding the different tiers of coverage. How will they understand their choices relative to prevention and co-pays? In addition, wellness and prevention programs are built into some of the health care reform legislation. Will those have disparate outcomes relative to health literacy, or for vulnerable populations in general? Paasche-Orlow replied that the planning committee for HARC 2010 has heard requests to make health reform part of the discussion.

Intrigued by Cooper's long list of potential collaborators, Isham suggested including systems engineers, those working on decision support, decision science, process flow analysis and design, and quality improvement science. It may be, he said, that academic settings are themselves disadvantaged with respect to state-of-the-art technical processes and support. Cooper agreed that there is a need to reach beyond academia. To really understand what is going on and what resources are available, one needs to go to the places where people are delivering care and to the communities where the target audience lives. Schillinger also agreed, adding that Larry Green from the Centers for Disease Control and Prevention (CDC) used to say, "It is not just about putting research into practice, but practice into research." That ideal was part of the genesis of the practice-based research networks supported by Agency for Healthcare Research and Quality (AHRQ). Merely studying things in one's own backyard is not representative of how the world is moving. There is tremendous variation in practice settings, even within a practice-based research network.

Paasche-Orlow added that the field is calling for dismantling the silos in which researchers live and work to involve more people. One of the keynote speakers for next year's HARC meeting is Nicole Lurie, who served as the chair of IOM's Roundtable on Health Disparities and is someone who interacts with both academia and the real world.

Rima Rudd, from the Harvard School of Public Health, sees the need to bring new people to the table. The first 10 years of health literacy research focused on the patient: the patient cannot read well; it is the patient's fault. Research is finally looking in the mirror at our providers' communication skills and at the broader context, as Schillinger noted. Where are the openings within the health care system to make changes and begin focusing on the system and the context? Schillinger said that an example of a system change is the role that health literacy can play in reducing hospital readmissions. The discharge program at Boston Medical Center has shown the great impact that health literacy can have in this area. Given that with health reform, institutions lose money if patients are readmitted, health literacy system interventions have a real opportunity to show benefit.

Cooper responded with two examples. First, a clinical psychologist pointed out that health literacy researchers act as if there is good understanding of what is going on, but that is not true. Health literacy research needs to include experts from psychology, neuropsychology, and psychometrics in order to answer such questions as, what makes a person have difficulty understanding and processing information? It is not as simple as completing a checklist of words. Second, within organizational culture, there is a need for measurement of how health systems work, how teams work, and how the culture of an organization influences the way care is delivered. The health disparities field, as Schillinger mentioned, has moved into a socioecological framework, bringing in communities and using participatory approaches in order to increase understanding of and benefit to the community populations. Involving those who understand more about measuring environmental context and social environment as well as physical environment and social policies will enhance the quality of health literacy research.

Betsy Humphreys, roundtable member from the National Library of Medicine (NLM) suggested that library information science be added to the list of collaborators because of their knowledge of information seeking behavior and information delivery. Through its work to connect people with good health information, the NLM has learned two things. First, some information services have to be adjusted for vulnerable populations. But sometimes the services are fine, the user just needs much more personal intervention to use the service; they need an explanation for why the information will be useful to them, what they can use it for, and when they should use it. A group of nonusers can become very happy users of existing services with just a personal intervention to help them figure out why.

Debra Roter of Johns Hopkins Bloomberg School of Public Health said she was concerned that the studies discussed, while providing insights, are not large enough to disentangle the confounding effects of ethnicity, culture, and literacy in the United States. The next step forward is to look across silos, she said, without forgetting that our public health mission is to reduce disparities and understand pathways and relationships. Paasche-Orlow agreed and said that in research that examines the effect of these variables on outcomes, there is a covariance problem. One can, for example, identify race bias of clinicians and there should be continued efforts to find things to do about environmental or institutional racism. The long term goal is to remove race bias from the medical care system, and that will take time. But what is the proportion of the variance that comes from race bias versus other types of things? It may be that race bias will be the important variable some time, but at other times it may not be as important.

Amy Wilson-Stronks, roundtable member from the Joint Commission, suggested articulating the research in terms of what it means for practice. There are some practices that are known to improve outcomes, such as access to language services, but despite the evidence, these practices are not implemented.

Isham ended the discussion session by asking whether researchers tend to cluster their studies in some areas more than in others because those areas are easier to study or better thought through. Is the research portfolio distributed appropriately? Do researchers intend to produce practical knowledge that people can do something about in the short run? Would there be value in prioritizing areas and taking on some tough questions? It seems that the complexity of the health care interface is less well understood as a contextual factor, but it provides a real opportunity for some interventions, for example, mammography rates among vulnerable populations may go up by having same-day mammography available at the clinic. Are the questions being studied prioritized by the likelihood of producing something that can be acted upon?

Schillinger replied that Isham's approach is an evidence-based and rational approach to inquiry. Yet research is more opportunistic, based on the principal investigator's expertise. Those with a background in communication will study literacy. There may be opportunities for professional development there, said Paasche-Orlow, adding that funding sources set the agenda as well. Setting priorities is a good idea, Cooper added, but it must be done within the broader setting including environmental issues. Other disciplines and expertise need to be at the table. Schillinger pointed to Michael Wolf's work on the complexity of the pill bottle; it involved basic science all the way to policy change.

4

The Role of Health Literacy in Health Information Technology

HEALTH LITERACY AND MEANINGFUL USE OF HEALTH IT

Joshua Seidman, Ph.D.
Meaningful Use, Office of Provider Adoption Support
Office of the National Coordinator for Health Information Technology

The meaningful use of health information technology (IT) has a role to play in reducing health disparities. There are challenges posed by health disparities and barriers around health literacy, but there are potential solutions. When the American Recovery and Reinvestment Act passed in February 2009, it included a set of incentives around the meaningful use of health IT.[1] Congress provided money for adoption as well as money for the meaningful use of health IT to improve the quality, safety, and efficiency of healthcare.

Meaningful use is not about technology. Technology is the tool, but meaningful use is about improving health and transforming health care. There are three stages of meaningful use. The first stage is focused on data capture and sharing. This first stage can help in understanding health literacy. Stage two focuses increasingly on advanced care processes. Stage three focuses on improving outcomes. The Health Information Technology for Economic and Clinical Health (HITECH) Act of 2009 established a federal advisory committee that will make recommendations to the Department of Health and Human Services (HHS). The recommenda-

[1] See http://www.hhs.gov/recovery/.

tions become a series of objectives and measures. A notice of proposed rulemaking was issued in January 2010.[2]

Health literacy is important to each of the five outcome priorities established by the health IT policy committee. These outcome priorities are to

1. improve quality, safety, efficiency and reduce health disparities;
2. engage patients and families in their health care;
3. improve care coordination;
4. improve population and public health; and
5. ensure adequate privacy and security protections for personal health information.

It is clear that health literacy is relevant to the first priority, which specifically aims at reducing health disparities. But health literacy is also relevant to thinking about how health information is used to reach the goals of engaging patients and families, improving care coordination, and improving population and public health. Public hearings are being held on these priorities. The first public hearing, on patient and family engagement, was held in April in Washington, DC. HHS is accepting public testimony at the hearings, but there is also a Federal Advisory Committee blog[3] for input from the public. All comments become part of the public record.

A series of themes has emerged from the first hearing and the blog. Each has implications for creating information for patients that truly addresses their health literacy needs. The following are the list of themes:

- Provide real-time patient access to data
- Incorporate patient-generated data into EHR
- Encourage innovation
  - —Connect home and community to care delivery settings
  - —Consider a bold initiative (e.g., 50 percent of care rendered at home)
- Create sense of community among patients and with health team
  - —Achieve 4 *E*s: engage, educate, empower, and enable
  - —Meet needs of diverse population
- Focus more on patient outcomes measures versus traditional process measures
- Engage with the public about meaningful use
  - —Consider reorienting meaningful use criteria to what is meaningful to patients

---

[2] Final rules were issued in July and can be found at http://www.hhs.gov/news/press/2010pres/07/20100713a.html.

[3] See http://healthit.hhs.gov/blog/faca/.

Health literacy is an important part of the theme, "creating a sense of community among patients and with the health team," especially when thinking of the four E's: engage, educate, empower, and enable. Patients need information they can understand, use, and act upon.

A June 4 hearing focused on using health IT to eliminate health disparities, with a strong emphasis on solutions. The first of three panels covered health literacy and data collection, the second was on cultural issues including language, and the third was on access—to health care, health information, and technology. Panelists considered several questions: What are the greatest risks of health IT implementation in increasing disparities? What innovations can prevent these risks? What research can guide health IT implementers? What patient/family engagement strategies can help support future meaningful use of health IT? How can meaningful use of health IT reduce disparities? What health IT applications can improve literacy, access, cultural relevance of health information?

While considering strategies to pursue, it is clear that ignoring technology is not a viable strategy. There are challenges in accessing technology, one of which is that it may create additional barriers and increase disparities. This is a real concern, and HHS is very focused on the potential, unintended consequences of evolution of health IT in this country. But that should not prevent forward movement because barriers can be overcome.

Ethnographic observations are critical for identifying needs, Seidman said. When he was a board member of a transitional house for homeless women who needed help becoming self-sustaining, the women asked for a computer in the house so they could become fully active participants in society. With the computer, they were able to obtain some basic computer skills, which helped them get jobs.

When spending time with populations that might use a technology, it is important to meet people where they are. Providing information in writing may not be the answer; maybe audio or video is a better approach to use. One must think about different ways to deal with health literacy barriers than have been used in the past. A young child who needs to learn how to use an asthma inhaler might learn better watching a video of himself being taught to use it than reading written instructions.

EHR-generated data can help with tailoring health information. Data collected through the EHR—through health risk assessment, biometrics, remote monitoring—can improve understanding of how to target information to a person's individual needs at a particular moment in care. Health literacy is an important part of this targeting.

Making data available in real time for patients is another important theme that emerged from the patient-family engagement hearing. It is important to think about not increasing disparities when determining how to implement an EHR. According to Seidman, Neil Calman[4] found lack of trust and respect to be a tremendous barrier to sharing data with patients. However, when exam rooms were designed for a more trustful and respectful relationship between patient and clinician, the two could view the EHR together. When the data in the record are shared in this way—either in the exam room or through a portal in the home—it potentially changes what is in the record and how it is written. Strategies are needed for translating clinical administrative data into lay terminology.

Seidman encouraged participants to visit the Health Information Technology Website[5] and post to the federal advisory committee blog. All comments are entered into the public record and help shape how meaningful use deals with issues of health disparities.

PROMOTING HEALTH LITERACY VIA INNOVATIVE HEALTH TECHNOLOGIES

Michael Wolf, Ph.D., M.P.H.
Feinberg School of Medicine
Northwestern University

How can health IT deliver health information to patients and families, streamline and standardize health care practices, and continuously connect with patients in order to simplify health system demands? Health education is not a one-time endeavor, nor is connecting with patients to support their role and responsibilities in health care. Can health IT help to continually and systematically connect patients to what they should do to manage their health? What are the range of uses one might envision for various health technologies in the context of the health literacy response?

First, what does health IT encompass? The IOM report (2004) pointed out the health system's complexity as a target for intervention. Health IT can include using telephones to monitor disease (Schillinger et al., 2008). Electronic health records are increasingly popular, not only as a support for quality care, but also to promote patient education in a timely manner. The Internet is a valuable source of information, but such use requires some sort of rating for people to know which health information is accurate and easy to understand. Interactive video and games are especially good technologies for kids. The Centers for Disease Control and Prevention's (CDC) website has many sophisticated games for teaching self-

[4] Neil Calman is President and Chief Executive Officer of the Institute for Family Health.

[5] See healthit.hhs.gov.

management of asthma and other chronic diseases. Handheld devices, such as cell phones, smartphones, and iPads deliver health education. Medical devices enable home monitoring, sending real-time information back to a provider. And finally, computerized agents enable tailoring of information to the needs of the patient at discharge (Bickmore et al., 2010). Health IT can be based anywhere; in hospitals and clinics, pharmacies, schools, public libraries, workplaces, and patient homes.

Health IT can be used for many purposes, including

- conveying patient information and promoting behavior change,
- eliciting patient issues and concerns and for screening,
- monitoring chronic disease,
- standardizing clinical protocols,
- tracking patient progress and outcomes, and
- prompting related health care provider behavior.

Through health IT, one can expand the target audience, tailor tools as needed to the individual, deliver information in a timelier manner, standardize the message, and layer content for patients who want to dig deeper using videos, interactive technologies, and websites. Processes of care can be automated. Resources can be delivered more efficiently and tools can be more sustainable.

There is potential for cost savings as well, Wolf said. Imagine that a patient comes into a general internal medicine practice and is led to an exam room and his or her vitals are taken by a nurse. The nurse identifies the patient through the EHR as being eligible for colon cancer screening. The patient watches a brief video before the doctor visits because time motion studies have revealed that short, brief educational tools fit within that space before the doctor enters the room. The doctor does not have to worry about what to tell the patient about colon cancer screening. The focus is more on the decision making and coming to a resolution. The patient can then be handed a print tool with tangible information generated so the patient can review the content that was discussed with images and language mapped to what they saw in the video.

Even in offices that do not have EHRs, such as federally qualified health centers, there are ways to help with chronic disease management. For a Missouri Foundation for Health study, Wolf's team worked with a Microsoft Office package to give practices basic tools to flag patients who need diabetes education and to help with tracking and follow up. One has to work within the confines of a practice—what is available for it and what its patients are able to use.

In addition to benefits, there are also incredible constraints, Wolf said, especially working with lower literate populations. These constraints include not only patient access and skills, but also provider access and skills. Patients often need new skill sets to interface with health IT; can they navigate a website, can they interact with the EHR patient portal? For providers, how is the practice changing and what are patients being asked to do? Is the clinical environment ready to change? In the Missouri Foundation study, asking staff to obtain new skills was very difficult.

Another constraint may be communication barriers between IT systems. Health care systems use different electronic health platforms that may not always translate one to another, or from a medical system to a pharmacy system. On some systems, such as Microsoft's HealthVault, a personal health record includes not just health care provider information, but also patient-entered information, which has to be kept up to date by the patient. Finally, automating certain patient or provider processes may be beneficial in terms of streamlining care, but the risk is that people become dependent on the tools. They think things are happening, when in fact, they may not be.

One constraint is illustrated in a recent study of 131 low-income adults (Jensen et al., 2010). Those with low health literacy skills reported less Internet use (e.g., email, search engines, and online health information seeking), and differences were mediated by age. A larger study showed patients with more limited cognitive abilities, less education, and older age showed greater anxiety with adoption of new technologies (Czaja et al., 2006). In another study it was found that, regardless of education and prior computer experience, the majority of older adults struggled when asked to go onto a Medicare website to try to perform some basic information retrieval (Czaja et al., 2008). The Internet can be an incredibly effective tool for many, if not most patients, but more user testing is needed, along with much more research on how best to design Internet tools and to make the interface accessible for all patients across literacy skills.

Efforts to develop effective and sustainable chronic disease self-management tools can run into trouble if the tool does not meet the practice's needs, for example, putting a kiosk with one educational tool on colorectal cancer screening in a center when that tool only meets the needs of 10 percent of the practice. Even low-tech strategies are a challenge without additional financial resources, ongoing IT support to deal with problems that occur, and a champion who can influence the practice to make sure it is implemented. Even a prescription label, designed and tested, was found, once it was moved into a pharmacy software system, to have many limitations that prevented making all the changes desired. A switch was made to a different system, with fewer limitations, but the example illustrates how each system has its unique barriers.

From a systematic literature review conducted with the Foundation of Informed Medical Decision Making, Wolf reviewed 21 studies comparing multimedia with print tools in terms of effectiveness, regardless of whether the outcome was education, decision making, instilling attitudes, or promoting a health behavior change. It does matter, however, if the outcome is procedural versus declarative. Video might be better for showing how to use an asthma inhaler. But for declarative content, such as learning the basic facts about asthma, print materials may be better because they offer an opportunity for repeated review. There is a value in video and print, especially when it is integrated. Having a tangible tool supports learning with video. Add video if there is a good reason, not just because it is snazzy, Wolf said.

In the context of promoting good health through health IT, standardization is important. Several studies examining how EHRs have uploaded physician instructions for medication have found problems. System breakdowns include unnecessary variability across different health systems (Bailey, 2009) and poor translation in pharmacy software and language access (Sharif and Tse, 2010). Many of the systems have been automated, yet there is incredible variability and poor quality because they are using insufficient health technologies to perform the translations. Some use web-based browsers that can provide inaccurate language or inconsistent information.

Problems can occur with e-prescribing, and data can be lost. It becomes difficult for an EHR to obtain good quality data on medication adherence, for example, if some patients are paying out of pocket for generics. The information is not being captured. When thinking about developing health IT systems, one must also think about the limitations in the use of health IT. Continuous quality improvement means health technology designers have to be aware of how the providers and patients will be interacting with the technology.

When thinking about health IT, there are several things to consider, Wolf said. Comprehensive evaluations are needed to assess not just the impact, but the fidelity of the rollout of health technologies to promote health literacy. The effects by age and literacy level are important to examine. Cost must be assessed and researchers must ask if using health technology will increase disparities. Will health IT be accessible or will it disenfranchise places that serve the most vulnerable populations? Critically consider use of new technologies. The iPad might be the new thing, but will it be around for awhile? Finally, seek to improve IT linkages across systems.

DISCUSSION

Isham began by asking about the impact of the iPad, cell phones, and smartphones on the issues of access and health literacy. Wolf replied that there are many studies on the use of cell phones and monitoring devices for patients with HIV and medication adherence. There are several iPhone applications that would probably translate to an iPad application to help patients. iPill is a medication management tool worth examining in this way. None have been fully evaluated in any context. It would be interesting to see how people would use it and what the cost-effectiveness is.

William Ross, roundtable member from Washington University said he has seen vulnerable patients who are very willing to watch a video while waiting for an appointment in his nephrology practice. But is there a way to standardize approaches? Wolf responded that the key is evaluation and process outcomes. How are people using the technology? How do they want to receive information? Approaches vary widely. Some send audio messages through iPads even though research shows that audio messages alone are one of the most ineffective methods in terms of retention of education messages. Others send text messages, although the effectiveness of that approach is not known. Because of their efficiency, using many technologies may be a good thing to get the messages across.

Rather than standardization, Seidman said his group is interested in disseminating best practices. HHS has grants with 60 regional extension centers around the country along with a health IT research and resource center that helps identify and share best practices to build communities of practice around what works and what does not. These centers share the leading examples of how to use various technologies for meaningful use of health IT.

When asked how meaningful use in health IT can address literacy and culture, how it can be incorporated into rule making, Seidman replied that, without commenting on the final rule, he would like to see more sharing of what is being done, how technologies are being used to deliver patient-specific education resources that are tailored to individual needs. It would be valuable to determine how to communicate and use that experience as a guide for the rest of the industry. Through other grants and contracts, HHS is looking for ways to stimulate innovation by understanding consumer needs. HHS also has contracts through extension programs to learn how EHRs are being used for patient-family engagement strategies. He expects to see a series of case studies and best practices generated. The regional extension centers are serving small practices and safety net providers.

Scott Ratzan, roundtable member from Johnson & Johnson, reflected on all the technology opportunities that have arisen in the past 20 years, most recently the wireless technologies. Mobile phones have penetrated deeply, even into vulnerable populations. The launch of Text4Baby with the White House was an innovative partnership. But it is still unclear how to determine the number of people who are getting the information and making health behavior decisions that are appropriate. What can the roundtable do to foster information sharing and help with discussions on disparities? The IOM has several groups on disparities, communications, health literacy, quality. It is time to foster the next steps.

Seidman called for more integration of technologies into the care delivery system. Studies clearly show that patients still want to get information from their personal clinician. Could something like Text4Baby be integrated into the EHR and create an interface so one of those messages goes to the consumer, but also is shared with the provider and entered into the record? What parts of the record can be used to better target and tailor messages that go to the patient, such as those in Text4Baby? He added that the meaningful use workgroup of the health IT policy committee is discussing integration and targeting of messages as part of the stage two and stage three meaningful use objectives, attempting to set expectations at increasingly higher levels without dictating exactly what should be done so that room for stimulating innovation and creativity remains.

When asked about the use of videos for patients, Wolf described the importance of evaluating the protocol in the clinic setting, examining each step in the process, determining how patients move in and out of the clinic, and the different roles of the providers that are touch points for the patients. Such an evaluation can result in substantial change in what is actually done. For example, in a study on medication therapy management, the original idea was to involve nurses in the reconciliation process. But it was found that was not needed. Whether it is using a patient education video or changing a process to ensure a patient and a clinician talk together, it is important to evaluate what is happening.

Isham made several comments. First, health literate IT programs are those that are designed so that the default options are the norm, as opposed to having to put together a series of activities that require winding one's way through a maze of steps and technology in order to do the right thing. This is the design principle that should be used in developing EHRs. Second, in thinking about applications being designed for direct consumer use, it seems that the current health IT design assumes a simple illness that is complemented by in-person care. Such systems do not take into account the illness complexity of many patients. Finally, in encouraging innovation in health IT it is important to provide incentives and determine meaningful use, but it is equally important not to stifle innovation.

Paasche-Orlow said he hopes to see innovation that pushes providers to change how they are using EHRs. Right now EHRs are used to protect the business model and defend the movement of data to make it hard for patients to get data moved from place to place. That must change, he said. There is too much emphasis on how the doctors use the EHR. The health literacy conversation brings into the discussion how consumers and other nondoctors are going to use these systems. Wolf said it is important to think as broadly as possible about the use of health IT. The current statutory authority focuses on the use of EHRs, and the leverage points are with Medicare and Medicaid providers. But in the long term, it is important to think much more broadly than this, he said.

5

Professional Development in Health Literacy Research

HOW DO WE BUILD THE FIELD OF HEALTH LITERACY RESEARCH?

David Baker, M.D., M.P.H.
Feinberg School of Medicine
Northwestern University

In discussing how to build the field of health literacy research, the first question to ask is, what should health literacy research look like in 2020? Twenty years ago, health literacy research was in the era of discovery and enlightenment because it was recognized that there were patients who could not read and understand the things expected of them in the health care setting. Next came the era of epidemiology and association when it was discovered that low literacy was associated with poor knowledge and self-management skills, underuse of preventive services, higher hospitalization rates, and increased mortality. Causal pathway research came next, pathways that went beyond reading ability alone. There is still a great deal of work needed to understand causal pathways. Most recently, research is moving to the testing of interventions. The HARC conference was exciting in its breadth of research on different types of interventions. Determining how to design and implement interventions will be long, hard, incremental work.

Better educational tools that can be integrated with routine care are needed. Delivery systems—personal health records, telephone, new media—must improve. Even if the tool is excellent, if the users are not interested or do not want to listen, the tool will not help them. A key challenge now is to identify ways to empower and activate patients.

To move health literacy research forward, there needs to be a broader multidisciplinary group of researchers working on the problem. Clinician-investigators are not the best group to be developing strong interventions; their strength is in developing strategies for implementing solutions into routine care. Cognitive psychologists and people from the learning sciences are needed to develop interventions. Strategies are needed to bring these groups together.

In terms of causal pathways, it is now recognized that worse health outcomes for individuals with low health literacy are not simply due to inability to comprehend print, multimedia, and oral messages. Causes are multifactorial, including differences in background knowledge, community beliefs and norms, information-seeking behaviors, self-efficacy, and healthcare seeking behaviors. To explore causation, there needs to be outreach to such fields as sociology and medical anthropology to understand health and healthcare beliefs, healthcare seeking behaviors, community norms, and social networks.

A study of hospitalization rates on 3,000 Medicare patients found that rates were about 30 percent higher for patients with low literacy (Baker et al., 2002). After tracking the patients for 7 years, age-adjusted mortality for people with low literacy was 52 percent higher than for those with adequate literacy (Baker et al., 2007). Clearly, there must be other factors besides the health care system that are affecting longevity. The focus needs to go beyond the healthcare system. To explore these causal pathways requires partnerships with researchers from other disciplines.

Fostering a diverse new set of investigators who can develop effective interventions requires better educational tools and systems, including more use of lessons from the learning sciences and cognitive psychology, Baker said. For implementation science, communication needs to be *hard wired* into the healthcare system. The question is not one of whether to use multimedia or print. It is about designing a system of integrated education and reinforcement of key messages that can be applied in everyday practice and meet patients' learning styles.

There are several avenues for bringing in other disciplines to health literacy research. HARC is one. A new summer institute, modeled after the American Heart Association's epidemiology conference or the National Institutes of Health's Office of Behavioral and Social Sciences Research summer research training conference, is another possibility. A summer institute could help junior investigators develop their knowledge and skill set. Applications could be required so that attendees come in with some level of preparation, and scholarships need to be provided.

Practice-based research networks offer a tremendous opportunity for partnerships to test practical health literacy interventions. The Health Resources and Services Administration (HRSA) is sponsoring a new network on comparative effectiveness called CHARN (Community Health Applied Research Network). There should be excellent partnership opportunities within CHARN for health literacy research. The health maintenance organization (HMO) research network is well established and is another resource to consider. The bottom line, Baker said, is that is it imperative to engage other disciplines if health literacy research is going to move forward.

HEALTH LITERACY RESEARCH: BUILDING THE FIELD

Debra Roter, Dr.P.H.
Johns Hopkins Bloomberg School of Public Health

The Institute of Medicine (IOM) has played an important role in developing the field of health literacy. Especially important is the IOM's introduction of the notions that health literacy is a function of literacy skills *in relation to* literacy demand. While health literacy research has grown exponentially, it has been largely from the vantage point of individual literacy skill assessment and deficit amelioration, somewhat in regard to measurement and reduction of literacy demand, but with almost no attention to the *in relation to demand* pathway pioneered by the IOM report.

The focus of her presentation, Roter said, is a critical address of the state of the art. Is the field of health literacy theoretical enough to be creative? And is it creative enough to flourish?

Beginning with the notion of theoretical creativity, there is nothing as theoretically interesting as a good question; to ask the right question requires logic, intuition, and curiosity as well as background and grounding in experience. And to do this well, to keep the research question useful and relevant, is to partner with natural constituents. We cannot have confidence in the questions asked if they are asked in isolation of those who are most directly affected by the answers. The application of community-based participatory research is critical in this light because it challenges researchers to be honest. Silos exist across academic disciplines, as well as between community groups and the researchers, with the result of insulating the field and limiting its relevance. Far too frequently, participatory collaborations are missing from health literacy research. Especially lacking have been partnerships between health literacy experts and those working in adult basic education and English as a second language (ESL) groups, with the formal education system, and with health delivery systems. These types of partnerships hold the promise of mutual benefit, and provide a source of creative—and theoretical—thinking.

Roter said she was going to suggest something quite heretical. All too often, formal theory can, paradoxically, act to constrain theoretical thinking. Theory can come from experience, observations, or the desire to reconcile conflicting empirical results. It need not be restricted to the handbooks of usual theory that proliferate on library shelves. Much research that is considered atheoretical is actually grounded in theory (formal or informal), but investigators, particularly young investigators, may lack the confidence to explicitly link their rationale and logic to hypotheses and predictions. More exploration and deliberation of this type is needed, and new and fresh eyes may be the ones that see the patterns and connections that previously misled.

An argument can also be made for health literacy to be more methodologically imaginative. Is it possible to investigate questions in ways that step outside the box? For instance, simulations have not been widely used in literacy research, but they can accomplish training, evaluation, and research objectives not possible in natural settings. Simulators can be patient proxies, including standardized, simulated, analogue, and virtual patients. Simulated or standardized patients refer most often to healthy people, or patients afflicted with a medical condition, who have been trained to accurately and consistently present a scripted case, or in some instances, provide improvisations and spontaneous role-playing while staying in character. Another type of simulator is an analog patient. These are untrained subjects recruited on the basis of specified criteria, for instance, a person with a family history of cancer, or someone who has recently visited a health clinic or received a particular diagnosis. The subjects are instructed to imagine that they are patients depicted in a videotape, audiotape, computer program, or written vignette. Often the viewed scenario has been experimentally manipulated in some way.

There is a great advantage to using simulations, especially for investigating unusual or logistically difficult phenomena or stressful, private situations within the medical context. As John McKinley noted, it is time for us to move into second and third generation methodologies that allow for experimental manipulation to disentangle confounded phenomena, such as ethnicity and literacy (McKinlay et al., 1996). In this vein, Roter said she and her colleagues used a combination of simulation and analog studies to investigate how genetic counseling is delivered. Two hundred genetic counselors interviewed simulated patients. This is by far the largest study of genetic counseling practice (Roter et al., 2007, 2009). The study found that genetic counselors who communicate in a way that is characterized as carrying high literacy demand, using grammatically complex language, are not liked very much. The simulated patients in these sessions were not satisfied with informational or interpersonal behavior of the genetic counselors. Moreover, analogue patients with restricted literacy were not able to recall as much from these high literacy demand sessions as they could from sessions that were more conversational.

Another creative methodology is the use of virtual reality to explore the likely response of patients to a variety of manipulated variables. It is known that analogue patients viewing computer-generated physicians act very much like patients in clinics. This line of research can shed light on the complicated domains by which cognition and emotion are communicated and also contribute to our understanding of pathways that relate to the *"in relation to"* component of the IOM definition of health literacy mentioned at the beginning of this talk.

The answer to the question, is the field of health literacy theoretical enough to flourish, may be tied to the extent to which we can meaningfully cross silos that foster innovative thinking, new methodologies, and authentic partnerships, Roter concluded.

DISCUSSION

Brach commented that her perspective of the presentations by Baker and Roter is that Baker focused on how to mentor and grow the field of health literacy research with new personnel while Roter focused more on the nature of research. Brach suggested that both approaches are needed in order to attract more young researchers and build a robust core of people doing health literacy work. Baker agreed: young researchers will be attracted by an interesting, exciting area that pushes the envelope in terms of methodologies. If a summer institute taught the most exciting, cutting-edge work it would be a draw. Roter suggested that this is an opportunity to create something transdisciplinary and integrative. Include an anthropologist, economist, clinical psychologist, and behaviorist at the table, she said. People will learn new ways of thinking and looking at the problem. Build something exciting and intellectually challenging, and young researchers will want to come. But it needs to be funded.

Yolanda Partida, roundtable member from the University of California San Francisco Fresno Center for Medical Education & Research, asked if there is a way to encourage practitioners to start thinking this way now. Baker replied that there are no good models yet. Take, for example, EHRs. Most practitioners still use paper records. But the technology problems with EHRs will be worked out. That will be time to engage those networks, to find out what are best practices, and to disseminate that information.

Rima Rudd offered that the way forward is to move outside the doctor's office. Most health activities take place at home, at work, in the community. Both presentations, however, were focused on the health-care setting. She challenged the presenters and other researchers to envision research questions that move the discussion out of the realm of the clinician's office and into the field of health literacy, which is community based and outside the very narrow clinical encounter. Baker agreed with the need to move beyond the clinical encounter to include research both pre- and post-encounter. Some researchers have begun this work in the area of obesity research and behavioral change research, but the focus must be on a continuum, not just one episode of care. Another point is the need for communication about health to begin early in schools. For example, people should not graduate from high school unless they know what diabetes is. Finally, the public health messages need to be the same as what people hear in the clinics, Baker said. Familiar messages in familiar language with familiar images, otherwise there is cognitive dissonance.

6

A Call to Action

THE NATIONAL ACTION PLAN TO IMPROVE HEALTH LITERACY

Cynthia Baur, Ph.D.
Centers for Disease Control and Prevention

The release[1] of the National Action Plan to Improve Health Literacy[2] (NAP) is a collaborative effort that began in 2003, with financial, moral, and intellectual support from several of the Department of Health and Human Services (HHS) agencies. Congratulations to all of the members of the HHS Health Literacy Workgroup for bringing this plan to fruition.

For a brief history, the Healthy People objectives were first launched in 2000,[3] which was the first time there was a national health objective on health literacy. Both the 2010 and 2020 updates[4] contain health literacy and related objectives. Healthy People was followed by the National Institutes of Health/Agency for Healthcare Research and Quality (NIH/AHRQ) program announcement to fund research, which was one of the first efforts to begin to establish the evidence base for health literacy as a major public health problem. The National Assessment of Adult

[1] See http://www.hhs.gov/ophs/news/20100527.html.
[2] See www.health.gov/communication/HLActionPlan.
[3] See http://odphp.osophs.dhhs.gov/pubs/HP2000/.
[4] See http://www.healthypeople.gov/.

Literacy[5] and the Institute of Medicine report (IOM, 2004) were both seminal events. 2006 is the year when those involved started to envision the need for a plan to pull everything together. The Surgeon General's office ran a 2006 workshop to examine the scientific basis for health literacy as a public health problem.[6] Many of the people at today's workshop presented at that event. Town hall meetings followed in 2007-2008 in four cities: New York City; St. Louis, Missouri; Sacramento, California; and Tampa, Florida. A draft plan was produced in January 2009 and the year was spent obtaining input from about 100 organizations. As one can see, a very participatory approach was used to develop the plan.

The vision articulated in the NAP holds a society-wide perspective on health literacy which is consistent with the IOM view (IOM, 2004). That vision is of a society that

- provides everyone access to accurate, actionable health information;
- delivers person-centered health information and services; and
- supports lifelong learning and skills to promote good health.

The plan also calls for a response from all sectors involved in health information and services. The plan has seven goals that relate to the notion that every sector has a role to play.

Those seven goals are as follows:

1. Develop and disseminate health and safety information that is accurate, accessible, and actionable.
2. Promote changes in the health care system that improve health information, communication, informed decision-making, and access to health services.
3. Incorporate accurate, standards-based and developmentally appropriate health and science information and curricula in childcare and education through the university level.
4. Support and expand local efforts to provide adult education, English language instruction, and culturally and linguistically appropriate health information services in the community.
5. Build partnerships, develop guidance, and change policies.
6. Increase basic research and the development, implementation, and evaluation of practices and interventions to improve health literacy.
7. Increase the dissemination and use of evidence-based health literacy practices and interventions.

---

[5] See http://nces.ed.gov/naal/.

[6] See http://www.surgeongeneral.gov/topics/healthliteracy/toc.html.

HEALTH LITERACY RESEARCH IN ACTION: EMPOWERING PATIENTS AND IMPROVING HEALTH CARE QUALITY

Carolyn Clancy, M.D.
Agency for Healthcare Research and Quality (AHRQ)

Today's release of the National Action Plan to Improve Health Literacy is something to be very proud of. It is clear from an AHRQ supported systematic review of all the studies done in health literacy several years ago (Berkman et al., 2004), that individuals with lower literacies have less health-related knowledge, increased incidence of chronic disease, poorer intermediate health markers, and less than optimal use of preventive health services. The report has been updated recently with 114 new articles, 13 that specifically address numeracy, and 33 that address interventions. The peer review draft of the update became available for comment on June 10.[7] The full report will be available in the fall of 2010.

Before we can address a problem, awareness of the problem must be very high. Collectively, we have done a good job of raising awareness. Addressing the public health problem of health literacy requires collaboration. Research should inform healthcare providers and facilities, public health officials, health communicators and educators, government agencies, producers of health and safety information, drugs, and devices; and payers and purchasers (including employers).

Let me share with you a personal experience of how my own awareness was raised. When I was a new health maintenance organization (HMO) doctor I gave my patients a simple form to fill out to gather information. To my surprise, many of the forms were returned unfinished or blank—because my patients were not able to fill them out. I learned that if the patients could not complete the form alone, we could do it together. It was easy to remedy the problem once I learned there was one. But it always shocks me to realize that had I not decided to use a form to collect information, I would not have known that some of my patients could not read.

Health literacy plays an important role in empowerment and healthcare quality. The recently passed Patient Protection and Affordable Care Act[8] creates an enormous space and opportunity that has not existed before. The National Action Plan furthers these transformational goals by calling for accurate, accessible, and most importantly, actionable information. How do we present information in a way that people not only understand, but know what they need to do next? This calls for improved

[7] See http://effectivehealthcare.ahrq.gov.
[8] See http://thomas.loc.gov/cgi-bin/query/z?c111:H.R.3590.as:.

communication, including informed decision making. Patients must feel they actually have a choice. Patient empowerment cannot happen unless there is an informed conversation where options are presented in an understandable way. It is this aspect of health care that is lacking in many settings. Increasingly, patients will need information about both the quality and cost of their options.

We face a long-term educational challenge as well as short-term challenges in identifying the interventions that can be evaluated and put in place right now. What kind of research is needed? We need research that goes beyond raising awareness that offers better measures of health literacy for more precise targeting of efforts to intervene. Those targeted interventions need to be evaluated. When an intervention is promising, work must be done to figure out how to disseminate it effectively. The one study that represents scalability and spread is the Michigan Keystone Project (Pronovost et al., 2006), which was about educating providers. Very few other interventions in health care have attained such widespread uptake of a successful intervention or program.

In terms of measurement, there needs to be expansion beyond literacy-based measures, Clancy said. For example, measures of health literacy that could be used on a telephone survey would create huge research opportunities. Ultimately, we need to get beyond individual measures and create national and community population measures. It would be extraordinarily helpful to clinicians to have some sense of the prevalence rate, as they often do for other conditions. For example, how likely is it that people from a particular area will have difficulty understanding information? That is part of the proactive nature of health care that will be part of the transformation journey we are launching here.

For 15 years, AHRQ has been in the business of supporting development of patient experience of care surveys, namely the Consumer Assessment of Healthcare Providers and Systems (CAHPS®). There is now a supplemental item set to help identify the patient's perspective on organizational health literacy. What is needed now are some specific health care quality measures to support quality improvement work.

It is very exciting that there were 33 published articles on intervention evaluations considered of sufficient quality to include in the latest systematic review. Yet the following are unanswered questions that urgently need to be addressed:

- How do we motivate patients to seek reliable health information and use it to make decisions?
- How do we overcome numeracy deficits in risk communication?
- What graphics enhance understanding?
- How do we effectively train practitioners?

- What are effective methods of teaching developmentally appropriate health curricula at each age?
- How do we make health systems easier to navigate?

In outpatient care, the average patient asks 1.5 questions from the time he or she arrives until leaving the office, and that includes questions about parking (Kaplan, 1991). It is very important to help people understand that their role has to be more participatory.

How do we get target audiences to embrace evidence-based practices? The good news in terms of improving care overall is that there is a growing list of promising practices, but they are not widely used. To foster widespread use requires collaboration with business people, with leaders of healthcare organizations, with consumer groups, and many others.

Taking health literacy interventions to scale requires that we answer some difficult questions. What kinds of tools are most helpful with which audiences? What economic arguments are persuasive? Health literacy interventions suffer from the same kind of challenge that many issues do. That is, it sounds good and it appears to be the right thing to do, but it is going to cost resources. Identifying that while there may be some upfront costs, there is likely to be savings in terms of such things as reduced readmissions or reduced problems in managing chronic illnesses is important.

How do we engage in effective partnerships with those outside the health system who have a profound influence on health literacy and outcomes? We have to think creatively about the universal pass-through points that can serve as the locus of health literacy interventions. Programs through churches have been successful, but only for people who go to church. What about more universal conduits, such as Verizon and the Department of Motor Vehicles? We have to expand our imaginations regarding community partners.

It is time to think about how to effectively implement interventions, Clancy said. An AHRQ-funded project called Project RED for reengineering discharge was developed at Boston University Medical Center. A randomized trial involved a nurse and a pharmacist giving patients focused attention at discharge and continuing follow-up with patients after discharge as an approach to reducing readmissions and emergency department visits (Jack et al., 2009).

The issue of potentially avoidable readmissions is high on policy makers' minds, as evidenced by the health reform bill. A new tool created for populations with lower health literacy may help. The Health Literacy Universal Precaution Toolkit[9] is a Web-based toolkit to help adult

[9] See http://ahrq.gov/qual/literacy.

and pediatric primary care practices implement health literacy measures. Produced for AHRQ by the University of North Carolina, it includes a six-step plan and 20 short tools to identify and address areas needing improvement. In the first few weeks after publication, it was downloaded nearly 9,000 times.

Researchers also must follow health literacy practices. AHRQ has developed the AHRQ Informed Consent and Authorization Toolkit for Minimal Risk Research.[10] The aim is to include low literacy populations in research and to ensure that consent and authorization is truly informed.

Where should we go from here? AHRQ supports user-driven research to answer questions that would-be users are asking and that involves would-be users in research design. This means going beyond the peer-reviewed article: creating tools and guides, writing trade press articles, training, leveraging opinion leaders, even pulling in Hollywood writers, since many people get their health information from television shows. It is important, Clancy said, that health literacy research makes a difference in peoples' lives.

HEALTH LITERACY RESEARCH: LOOKING TOWARD A NATIONAL AGENDA

Raynard Kington, M.D., Ph.D.
National Institutes of Health

The National Institutes of Health (NIH) fully supports the creation of this action plan. The foreword to the plan, written by Dr. Howard Koh, clearly articulates the need to advance our understanding of the problem of health literacy and the tools available to create health literacy interventions that will result in a positive way on the health of populations.

Since 2004, the NIH has had a program announcement focusing on understanding and promoting health literacy. It has been reissued three times; most recently in 2010. A wide cross-section of NIH institutes and centers signed on to support research under this RFA (request for application), as did AHRQ and the Centers for Disease Control and Prevention (CDC), our colleagues who have devoted so much attention to this topic. The goal was to encourage empirical research on health literacy concepts,

[10] See http://www.ahrq.gov/fund/informedconsent.

theory, and interventions, through mechanisms ranging from the standard R01[11] research grant to smaller R21[12] and R03[13] grants.

The specific objectives of program announcement PAR-10-133 included health literacy as a key outcome; health literacy as a key explanatory variable for some other outcome; methodological or technological improvement to strengthen research on health literacy; and/or prevention and/or intervention strategies that focus on improving health literacy. The scope is broad, from basic research to applied research, especially studies focused on incorporating individual, family, community, or health system and societal mediators of health literacy. Secondary analyses of existing datasets were also supported. A total of 77 grants were funded through the first two cycles for more than $64 million.

An analysis of 71 of those 77 grants shows that a majority were intervention studies (42 percent), followed by descriptive studies (30 percent), measurement and methods (25 percent), and a few basic mechanisms and pathways (3 percent). This illustrates a problem: we do not know enough about fundamental mechanisms that underlie the relationships between health literacy and a range of health outcomes. In addition to the programs funded through the program announcement, NIH supported an additional $218 million worth of research between 2002 and 2009, across an array of institutes and centers. These range from studies looking at the relationship between educational status and structure of the brain to interventions and dissemination research. This is more evidence of NIH's strong commitment and recognition of the relationship of health literacy to many of the goals that are part of our mission.

The NAP Goal 6—Research that supports basic behavioral research and the development, implementation, and evaluation of practices and interventions to improve health literacy—clearly represents a great opportunity for more basic research that will help in understanding fundamental, causal pathways. The NAP encourages behavioral research on several levels including the following:

[11] "The Research Project (R01) grant is an award made to support a discrete, specified, circumscribed project to be performed by the named investigator(s) in an area representing the investigator's specific interest and competencies, based on the mission of the NIH." (http://grants.nih.gov/grants/funding/r01.htm).

[12] "The R21 grant mechanism is intended to encourage exploratory/developmental research by providing support for the early and conceptual stages of project development." (http://grants.nih.gov/grants/funding/r21.htm).

[13] The R03 grant mechanism will support small research projects that can be carried out in a short period of time with limited resources." (http://grants.nih.gov/grants/funding/r03.htm).

- Identify and address gaps, such as numeracy and visual communication, in health literacy research.
- Develop more rigorous and comprehensive methods to measure individual and population health literacy skills that capture the full range of skills including listening and speaking, writing, numeracy, and cultural and conceptual knowledge.
- Develop methods to measure the full range of health literacy skills of health professionals and organizations.
- Explore technology-based interventions to improve health literacy.
- Develop and implement health literacy interventions based on theories and models—drawing from such related disciplines as communication, education, cognitive science, and medical sociology.
- Include health literacy measures in national and other surveys (ODPHP, 2010).

At NIH, this research is distributed across institutes and centers, but there is an effort to improve coordination and identify gaps for funding. OptNet opportunity network is providing more than $30 million to look at the broad topic of basic behavioral research. Not surprisingly in many areas of research, including this area, some basic issues of methods and measures are often a core part of the gap that is identified.

The NAP's Goal 7 focuses on increasing dissemination and use of evidence-based health literacy practices and interventions. The NIH is interested in doing a better job of translating research results for use in real-world settings. One of NIH Director Francis Collins' five priorities is to fund research that is relevant for health care reform. A big part of this priority is helping us disseminate the evidence we have so that it is more widely used across populations. The NIH has a long history of funding support in the area of dissemination and implementation research.[14] There is also an annual NIH conference sponsored by the office of Behavioral and Social Sciences Research that focuses on the science of dissemination and implementation. Health care reform and renewed interest in comparative effectiveness research make this work particularly important.

NIH is committed to funding research in health literacy, Kington said, and sees it as an essential part of facilitating the translation of advances in basic research into improvements in health in real-world settings. Increasing our investment in dissemination and translation will help ensure that the evidence we support is actually used.

[14] See http://grants.nih.gov/grants/guide/pa-files/PAR-10-038.html; http://grants.nih.gov/grants/guide/pa-files/PAR-10-039.html; http://grants.nih.gov/grants/guide/pa-files/PAR-10-040.html.

DISCUSSION

Arthur Culbert, roundtable member from Health Literacy Missouri, which hosted one of the town meetings in St. Louis, expressed excitement about the NAP. Because there is a great deal of activity in health literacy, he said, several states (Iowa, Minnesota, Wisconsin, Arkansas, and Missouri) have come together to form Health Literacy USA. The aim is to leverage efforts and move forward to put this National Action Plan into use within each state. Health Literacy USA can serve as a model for getting the important health literacy research onto the streets.

With a focus on practicality and measuring impact at the community level, Ross asked if tools such as Consumer Assessment of Healthcare Providers and Systems (CAHPS) have been validated at the community level and whether its use could be expanded. Brach responded that CAHPS has been rigorously developed in terms of cognitive and psychometric testing, but it has not been tested at the community level as a lever for change and improvement. Groups are beginning to use health literacy CAHPS, and AHRQ has a project to further investigate the use of CAHPS in improving and measuring quality improvement in the primary care practice. AHRQ is accepting applications on a rolling basis.

Ratzan suggested the need to look beyond clinical health literacy. That is to expand the focus from one of health being delivered in the health care setting to health being delivered in the societies in which people live. How do public–private partnerships fit in to this, he asked, and where does the funding need to come from? Where are the foundations and other parts of society that will be important? The advances in public health have not all come from government-driven systems but are often driven by private foundations. He challenged the group to devise a framework to foster public—private partnerships for health literacy, involving payers and providers, as well as private companies.

Baur responded that a formal partnership structure has not been highlighted in the NAP, but that the efforts of Health Literacy USA could be viewed as one type of such effort. That is an example of how efforts in health literacy can go beyond what is in the NAP. Research and creativity should not stop with the publication of the NAP. Baur challenged organizations to take the NAP and use it as the framework to, for example, elaborate partnerships, which is covered in Goal 5. Brach agreed that there is no global partnership framework, but the NAP enumerates the partners that need to be included. AHRQ is working with private partners that are health plans, developing a health plan version of the health literacy CAHPS tool for them. Kington added that the NIH is very supportive of public/private partnerships, though there can be difficulties. In health literacy, at least there would not be fights over intellectual property as there are in some research fields. The NIH Foundation is another mechanism; CDC has a similar foundation. The goal is to facilitate public/private partnerships with industry, for example, in precompetitive space.

Dreyer added his congratulations, calling this a "great moment." He plans to use the NAP in conversation with American Academy of Pediatrics leadership to say, "This is where we need to begin." But the reality is that only five states and one or two health plans are excited about the National Action Plan. Professional organizations can play a role in changing behavior of physicians and health care providers too. What are the plans for engaging them and what can the roundtable to do help, Dreyer asked. Brach acknowledged the limitations of working with one partner at a time. AHRQ is trying to make health literacy a part of everything it does. It is trying to feed tools to empower partners to move forward, whether they are visiting the health care innovations site, downloading podcasts in Spanish for consumers, or looking at consumer guides. Baur added that each of the government agencies involved has its own constituencies to reach. She wants to explore how the roundtable can help get the word out so that each organization takes the NAP and uses it to inform its thinking and set priorities. She expects to be on call to offer technical assistance, give talks on the plan, and help create tools.

Sharon Barrett, roundtable member from the Association of Clinicians for the Underserved, asked if there are plans to work with those who produced the National Partnership for Action to End Health Disparities.[15] The two major plans that are looking at collaborations at the national, regional, and local levels could come together and coordinate their efforts. Baur replied that several agencies that are active in health disparities are represented in the NAP. Guadalupe Pacheco from the Office of Minority Health, HHS, is a member of the work group. There is a lot of cross-talk between health literacy and health disparities, and there have been conversations about proposing new objectives within the health communication/health IT (information technology) framework around health disparities and health literacy. Kington added that the NIH is in the next cycle of the NIH strategic plan for health disparities and minority health research and this area of research is clearly going to be part of that plan.

[15] See http://minorityhealth.hhs.gov/npa/.

7

Health Literacy Research Contributions to the National Action Plan

THE ROLE OF HEALTH LITERACY RESEARCH IN THE NATIONAL ACTION PLAN

Terry C. Davis, Ph.D.
Louisiana State University Health Sciences Center

Goal 6 of the National Action Plan calls for the expansion of the size and scope of health literacy research and evaluation. Nineteen strategies are provided for research teams, program evaluators and funders. This goal raises several issues for consideration:

- How do we translate effective research findings into practice? Will they be implemented reliably? Are they sustainable?
- Do we understand why low literacy is related to worse health outcomes—is it more than knowledge, skills, capacity? What else is literacy a marker for?
- What is the economic impact of inadequate health literacy? What is the cost of low health literacy?
- What are the research opportunities and challenges?
- What is the role of health literacy research in health care reform? What are critical questions that feed into policy?

It is time to broaden our research focus to include strategies to translate proven interventions into action. Attention must be paid to the practical details, the "how-tos" of successful implementation and sustainability in real-world settings in different communities. Knowing the cost of the problem may help drive policy. Additionally, there is a need to drill down on issues that are not clear. For example, why is low literacy related to worse health outcomes? The impact of poverty, social disadvantage, and poor quality of care on outcomes has been documented, but what else is going on? What is health literacy a marker for? It is likely a key, but not the only key.

In addition, several crosscutting research themes offer exciting possibilities. These include health care redesign, health insurance reform, improving navigation and community-based participatory research, removing health literacy barriers to clinical trials, addressing disparities, health literacy measurement in national and other surveys, and pre K through 12th and adult education and health education. Davis said that one of her long-standing concerns involves the pervasive national problems with K-12 education. Currently it is estimated that 30 to 40 percent of sixth graders will not graduate from high school. The markers are known—school attendance, behavior, scores, and grades. These children need more than better health literacy. Evidence is emerging that student achievement improves if there are high expectations, impassioned teaching, provision of better reading and math skill building, more practice, and a lot of support. Attention to this challenging problem will also help address the health literacy of future adults and families.

Crosscutting research themes are interesting opportunities, but are crosscutting agendas possible? And if so, who will be the responsible agency? The bureaucracy of research makes collaborations difficult. Funding is offered largely by disease, and researchers most commonly function and publish in silos.

The good news is that health literacy research is evolving. The field has finally moved beyond assessing readability and individual literacy. Self-management interventions have moved beyond knowledge transfer to include patient behavior, support, and empowerment. Areas where work is still needed include outcomes research and identifying methods to make health numeracy more user-friendly. For example, in outcomes research focusing on preventive services utilization, patients' completion of screening tests are most commonly self-reported and usually not tracked for more than 1 year. More longitudinal studies are needed. Another promising area is numeracy. Because of the work of Dr. Russ Rothman and others,[1] it is now clear that numeracy is a pervasive problem even among younger adults with adequate reading skills. Ameri-

[1] Dr. Russell Rothman and colleagues (2006) conducted a study that showed that those with low literacy and low numeracy skills have significant difficulties understanding food labels.

can adults do not perform well on math word problems; proficiency in this type of math skill is needed to understand and use food and drug labels and dose medicine correctly. What can be done to make health care math more understandable and usable? With National Institutes of Health (NIH) and Agency for Healthcare Research and Quality (AHRQ) support, cutting edge research is being conducted.

The Institute of Medicine (IOM), the Centers for Disease Control and Prevention (CDC), the Health Resources and Services Administration (HRSA), the Joint Commission, and the United States Pharmacopeia (USP) are increasing attention on this issue, and new initiatives are being developed. Many health care providers—in state health departments and public and private health care systems—now understand why health literacy is important, and they are eager to initiate programs. They are eager to initiate programs, yet they lack clear understanding on how to practically implement them. The new toolkits will help, but some practices need more than a toolkit. They need guidance on implementation—a navigator or a coach.

Putting health literacy research into practice has challenges. The Health Literacy Universal Precautions Toolkit designed to help health care practitioners learn how to communicate more effectively with their patients has 20 very practical tools. But can they be reliably implemented and sustained? Darren DeWalt, a coauthor of the toolkit, tested it in eight practices and found that even five tools were too many.

Another example of the challenges of implementing and sustaining research findings and guidelines in real-world practices can be found in research (funded by the Missouri Foundation for Health and the American College of Physicians Foundation) conducted by Dr. Michael Wolf on implementation of a diabetes self-management intervention,. In this ongoing study of nine Federally Qualified Health Centers (FWHCs) in Missouri, three clinics implemented their standard diabetes education and counseling. Three other clinics implemented a patient-centered health literacy intervention using a self-management guide book, action plan counseling, and telephone follow-up by a trained "diabetes champion" at the clinic. The final three clinics implemented the same interventions from a "diabetes champion" at Northwestern University in Chicago who provided the education, counseling, and follow-up by telephone.

The preliminary results are telling. In the Northwestern-supported group, 84 percent of patients received the health literacy intervention as planned. In the three clinics that implemented the health literacy intervention on-site, rates of patients' education, counseling and follow-up varied: 4 percent in one clinic, 38 percent in a second clinic, and 94 percent in the third clinic. The low rate occurred because the nurse in charge did not want to do it and was not personally incentivized to do it. The high rate occurred in a small rural clinic, with a nurse who was committed and impassioned by the idea and saw it as part of her mission, although no financial incentive or extra time was offered. This is a prime example of why research is needed on how to implement more consistently. Will health literacy changes last and evolve without the presence of an impassioned advocate? The final question this research evokes is, can health care innovations that are found to work in study clinics also work in non-study clinics?

Davis said her research and speaking engagements have taught her that health literacy is receiving attention in state health departments, local health care systems, and community clinics. Impassioned advocates at many of these sites have developed and implemented effective approaches, but they never get written up and published and, consequently, are not known. She has also learned that there are hidden challenges in working with rural and distant community clinics. Her experience, she said, taught her that

- Transition from research in academic university hospital settings to community participatory research requires a significant amount of time. Researchers must be flexible.
- Federally qualified health centers value service—they are not familiar with research.
- Usual care varies from clinic to clinic.
- Clinic implementation of research protocols can vary widely (an impassioned champion is needed).
- Physician turnover can be high.
- It is difficult finding qualified research assistants in rural areas.
- Off-site investigators must account for "research burnout" of clinic staff and research assistants.
- A short patient education video (2 min) may still not work in interventions. (A computer and private space is needed to show video and someone is needed to set it up. Additionally, some patients say they do not have time to view it.)

There are also measurement questions to consider, said Davis. For example, are health literacy assessments actually measuring *literacy*? Another important question is to ask whether patients clearly understand the questions that are developed from the researcher's perspective. Recently, when training research assistants, Davis played the role of a patient and answered questions read to her. When actually answering the questions, it became clear, she said, that she was not sure how to answer several of them—even those she had written. The differences offered in Likert choices sometimes seemed ridiculous and, after about 20 minutes, she lost interest and motivation to finish. Patients are likely to do the same. With long assessments patients may *wear out* and not carefully consider their answers. Other measurement issues to consider are the problems of tracking population health literacy. Is it possible and will comprehensive assessments stay current? Health literacy is dynamic. It keeps evolving as tasks and demands increase. Computer literacy, for example, will be added to the 2016 NAALS (National Adult Assessment of Literacy). Should health literacy include ability to use the Web to obtain, process, and understand health information and services?

Davis said the most central questions are as follows: Does the goal of improving health literacy amount to improving clinical and public health communication and care systems? Will more precise data collection and comprehensive assessment help change the way health care is communicated and delivered? Is health literacy context specific?

Life is dynamic—health care and health literacy are evolving. The number of prescription and over-the-counter drugs is growing rapidly and will continue to do so. Science and technology are moving fast. Consumers are increasingly responsible for their health care. Health literacy research must keep up, Davis concluded.

NATIONAL ACTION PLAN TO IMPROVE HEALTH LITERACY: GOAL 6, RESEARCH

Rima Rudd, Sc.D.
Harvard School of Public Health

Goal 6—Increase basic research and the development, implementation, and evaluation of practices and interventions to improve health literacy

Of the seven goals detailed in the *National Action Plan to Improve Health Literacy*, Goal 6 uniquely focuses on research and provides 19 agenda items and strategies for a research agenda that will contribute to our knowledge base and illuminate pathways to improved health literacy and better health. The National Action Plan responds to and builds on the recommendations of the IOM report, *Health Literacy, A Prescription to End Confusion* (IOM, 2004). The IOM committee that prepared that report noted that early research in what was then a nascent field of inquiry did, by 2003, establish links between literacy and health outcomes. However, the IOM report also highlighted several research weaknesses that needed attention and gaps that ought to be bridged as the field develops. The identified limitations in the early research in the health literacy field include a narrow focus on one of five literacy skills, on the clinical exchange, and on the skills of patients. The NAP provides a research agenda that considers these issues and offers recommendations that address a wider array of literacy skills and health activities and that calls for increased attention to intervention research.

Early health literacy studies focused on the reading skills of patients. Yet, educators speak of five related literacy skills: reading, writing, speaking, listening, and math skills (numeracy). A good deal of information provided to the public and to patients is indeed in written format on the printed page and on Internet websites. At the same time, the spoken word delivered through the radio and television and in the exchanges between clinicians and their patients or clients are of critical importance to public health and to health care. Furthermore, as Apter and colleagues point out (2008), math skills and numeric concepts are embedded in and needed for many health related activities. A broader understanding of the multiple components of literacy and most especially of speaking and listening skills will allow researchers to explore the exchanges so critical to public health and to clinical encounters. In addition, attention to basic math skills and numeric concepts such as *normal* or *risk* will enrich our understanding of barriers to action and to decision making.

Most of the studies in health literacy have focused on activities within health care settings. Many early studies focused on samples of patients in emergency departments of hospitals, and other studies focused on patients in consultations with clinicians for chronic disease management. These studies are of ongoing importance and have been central to the ability of researchers to link literacy skills and health outcomes. The NAP suggests that researchers now broaden the scope of inquiry to explore the myriad settings—home, work, community—where people take health-related actions. It is within these settings that people encounter health related products, messages, materials and tools, and where they daily make critical decisions. Expanding the scope and moving beyond, but not ignoring, the clinical encounter, brings health literacy into public health and public policy discourse around community health. Such actions may expand the research group as well and serve to bring in colleagues from education, health policy, environmental health, and occupational health studies.

At the same time, the narrow attention that health literacy researchers have given to the skills and actions of individuals needs to be expanded. Individuals function in multiple roles—as caregivers, as patients, as consumers, and as community members. Zarcadoolas (2005), for example, has long called for attention to health literacy in terms of civic engagement. Health literacy, in this broader arena includes, for example, community access to information about environmental degradation and the ability of groups and communities to make decisions and take action.

The 2004 IOM report also noted that literacy does not take place in a vacuum. If reading skills are to be tested, the demands of the text must be assessed as well. The NAP calls for research that illuminates the barriers that people face as they encounter unfamiliar vocabulary, unusual processes, complex facilities, and cumbersome forms and legal documents. Some of these impediments to action have been thoroughly studied. For example, well over 1,000 studies attest to the poor quality of written health information—whether on paper or on the computer screen. We know that increasing access to information means improving the rigor of our materials development and piloting processes. Multiple guidebooks, such as the Doak, Doak, and Root classic (2007), have long been available to provide insight into best practices and processes.

Other impediments have not yet been as carefully documented or studied. The call to action offers a needed emphasis on the importance of research into system-level barriers and facilitators. Here too, some work has set the stage for research studies. Rudd developed the notion of a health literacy environment and Rudd and Anderson (2007) provided an assessment process and tool. Building on this work, DeWalt and colleagues (2010) have developed and piloted a tool for identifying system level barriers in medical practice. This is now being widely distributed and broadly tested.

Furthermore, while the multiple measures of the health literacy skills of patients have been developed, tested, and applied, little has been done to test the communication skills of public health or health care professionals in health literacy studies. Here too, a firm foundation for such research is well established in the work of health communication researchers with their attention to provider–patient interaction as well as to the value and efficacy of question asking and the *teach back* method. Consequently, Harper and colleagues (2007), for example, reported on the integration of health literacy into medical curricula, drawing from the research findings of scholars such as Roter (2004) and Schillinger and colleagues (2004). However, more research is needed to study the links between these professionals' skills and health outcomes for patients with limited literacy skills.

Finally, the major gap identified in the IOM report has to do with guidelines and gold standards. Implementation studies remain scarce and are still sorely needed. The NAP calls for program evaluation studies to explore barriers related to health communication, health systems, and the effects of purposeful change.

The research agenda suggested by the National Action Plan calls for studies of oral communication skills, of math skills and numeric assumptions, of the practices and processes of health care, and of the communication skills of health professionals. It also asks that we turn our attention to the multiplicity of settings within which people take health-related actions. In so doing, the NAP is recommending a strategy that reduces barriers to information, to decision making processes, to action, to health care, and to community well-being.

The U.S. Department of Education's 1993 and 2005 reports of literacy skills among U.S. adults give evidence of the strong links between literacy and social factors (Rudd, 2007). Analyses of the distribution of health literacy indicate that health literacy is related to health disparities. Everything we talk about when speaking of literacy and disparities, alone or together, must meld with the powerful issues of social justice.

Health literacy research offers evidence of links between literacy skills and prevention, early detection, chronic disease management, informed choice, illness, and early death. Social justice will not allow us to wait for the education systems to improve literacy skills of the public. At the same time, logic will not allow us to attribute health outcomes to individuals' literacy skills alone. Literacy, as the 2004 IOM report noted, is an interaction between the skills of individuals and the demands of health systems. Barriers to information, to care, and to individual as well as community-level decision-making and action—contribute to untoward health outcomes. They must be identified and removed.

Policy makers need an evidence base for suggested change, Rudd said. There is already a strong foundation for some of these issues. For example, we know that there must be professional rigor applied to the development and delivery of health information. (Rudd suggested that it be made criminal to disseminate incomprehensible materials critical to health, to healthful action, and to health decisions.) We may well want literacy-related regulations that set standards for health and social service environments and institutions and literacy-related communication criteria for the testing and licensing of professionals. However, we cannot move this agenda ahead without the research to provide insight into needed change and program studies to determine what actions prove efficacious. The National Action Plan offers more than a call—with strategies and links to examples, it illuminates a pathway, Rudd concluded.

DISCUSSION

One of the major things we are trying to improve, said Dreyer, is how the health care system communicates with patients and gives them information. The NAP says this needs to be measured. But how does one measure how a health system communicates? Davis agreed that is the crux. More work is needed on how to measure whether a health care system is designed for patients. Isham added that the system with its complexity is a key target. We need research and implementation tools for both the organizational level and environmental level of the health care system. As policy initiatives move toward the aggregation of the health care system, health literacy needs to keep pace by thinking about context and the degree of chaos and disorganization. How can the complexity be assessed, as opposed to the individual and his or her capabilities within the system?

Dreyer asked Rudd about her comments on regulations. How might regulations from the Centers for Medicare and Medicaid Services (CMS) and payment processes drive this? Rudd said CMS might mandate, for example, that patient education sessions be done in everyday language. *Knee* is such a better word than *patella*. Isham asked if researchers are the right people to redesign systems. Rudd responded that researchers, perhaps, should serve as evaluators rather than designers, which is reason to bring in the different skill sets discussed earlier.

Amy Wilson Stronks, roundtable member from the Joint Commission, called for mechanisms to make sure patients can provide information to providers so there is an exchange. The Joint Commission recently adopted new standards aimed at improving patient-centered communication through a larger project to advance effective communication, cultural competence, and patient- and family-centered care. Though not named, health literacy is a part of that. She asked Rudd for recommendations for the Joint Commission on ways to carry that forward to health care providers. Raising awareness and appreciation is the first step, replied Rudd. It is a profound literacy task to be able to take a feeling from within and be able to take that sensation and turn it into words for a stranger, or someone you see once a year. The challenge is to figure out how to make it easier for the person. Appreciating the task and then brainstorming solutions will reveal interesting possibilities that can be tested. And that means getting beyond the "smiley faces to frowning faces" scale to describe pain.

8

Lessons Learned from the Workshop

Isham suggested that the final session be devoted to a collective review of the day's presentations. To begin, this is a small research field, he said, and there is need for greater collaboration with disparities researchers. Furthermore, there is need for more connections with researchers in other disciplines who bring additional skill sets, as Lisa Cooper said in her presentation. A major question is, how can the field of health literacy research be expanded to add more people, as well as more scope and breadth of disciplines?

The presentations illustrated the two-sided nature of health literacy, Isham continued. One side involves the individual, with a focus on his or her skill set and capabilities, as well as how to prepare individuals to navigate the system. The other side focuses on the complexity of the system itself. This complexity is reflected in the need for clear communication, embedded communication, and process design. Coherent arguments were put forth about the need to standardize the process of care so that the system becomes less chaotic and provides more care. Standardization could incorporate the research lessons from health literacy on how to be more effective in approaching patients.

Another important point made today, Isham said, is that some hypotheses about health literacy are better developed than others. It is important to ask, he said, whether addressing some of these hypotheses will lead to usable and implementable interventions. Researchers will become involved if the work associated with a field is important and will make a difference. What is the mechanism at the front end to obtain input about the important problems? Is it the clinical part of the researcher's day that informs those questions? Is it the institution in which the researcher sits? Is there a way to look at a clinical problem in terms of consistently delivering excellent services to a broad population?

As the health care system becomes more sophisticated, with automated recording tools and processes, it inevitably leads to the conclusion that it is important to help individuals cope with the system and its output, Isham said. As the process and consistency of recommendations for delivering care improve, it becomes increasingly important to understand the issues of the patient, how he or she understands and communicates regarding these issues and the system. Health literacy is absolutely central to that, Isham stated. Profoundly understanding people's needs, preferences and values, and how science, health care, and medicine interface with those, is becoming more prominent.

The National Action Plan (NAP) is exciting and offers a coherent approach that will spawn a whole set of productive questions about next steps. It is a rich start for several conversations on implementing the plan, Isham concluded.

Culbert emphasized the role of the community, particularly, in the need for increased community-based participatory research so that the findings can be more easily translated back into the community. Ross called for a focus on the more vulnerable populations. Health literacy needs be viewed in a social construct, acknowledging the social and economic components, Ross said, which requires expanding the number of partners to include those in education, finance, health, and policy. Dreyer stated that thinking about disparities, health literacy, and the role of universal versus targeted interventions is key. Are there universal interventions that will be intensive enough to be given to all, or are targeted interventions the way to go? Do we know, he asked?

Rudd's discussion of the education system was particularly useful, Dreyer said. The education system is broken. When so many students do not learn math or writing or any of the other academic subjects, how can we expect them to learn anything about health? The NAP calls for teaching children from preschool through university about managing their own health. Are there specific interventions that can be used to promote education, he asked?

Barrett shared her appreciation for movement away from looking at an individual's deficits and moving to evaluate organizations and the environment in which health care delivery occurs. How can the health care system better communicate with patients? Other stakeholders need to be brought to the table; the silos need to come down. Health literacy should begin to disperse into the environment in which people live and work, broadening beyond the health care system.

Margaret Loveland, roundtable member from Merck & Co., said she was pleased to see the move from theoretical to practical; that community involvement is key and implementation skills are the place to focus. Furthermore, she said, the IT discussions were stimulating, especially the idea of using cell phones in an emergency to give crucial information such as how to use an inhaler or an asthma action plan. There were many good implementation ideas discussed, Loveland said.

Wong emphasized that social justice is a convergent factor around health literacy and health disparities. It is important to stop thinking about patients as passive recipients of care and to see them as actively involved in defining what care means to them. Consumers need to be empowered to proactively define their needs for maintaining their health, which in turn defines their core value systems. This has ramifications for examining the health care system, which is basically a sick care system. Under health care reform 30 million people who have been marginalized will be newly covered, resulting in tremendous social empowerment issues. It will be critical to not exacerbate disparities as the opportunity is presented to bring these individuals into the system, Wong said.

In terms of broad outreach or universal interventions versus focusing on vulnerable populations, Humphreys said she appreciated Schillinger's suggestion that programs be available for everyone, with more time and depth offered for people who need it. She also agreed with Isham on the need for a redesign of the process of health care. But the concern is that health IT will be implemented without redesign of health care processes. Designing health literate health IT systems can help. Ensuring greater access to better information for patients at the same time as providing better training for patients may be easier than redesigning the system once to accommodate health IT and then later redesigning it again to address health literacy issues. The National Library of Medicine's (NLM's) mission aligns nicely with the NAP goal of developing and disseminating health information that is understandable. NLM has a national network of libraries of medicine and connections with public libraries and other community organizations. There will be a lot of interest at NLM in building strategies that relate to its network and existing activities.

Wilson-Stronks said she gained understanding from the presentations on the need to collaborate, to break down silos, and to link multiple initiatives within organizations. Martha Gragg, roundtable member from Missouri Foundation for Health, said she is excited about sharing the NAP with the communities and organizations the foundation works with. She hopes the NAP will help in tracking what the foundation can affect and what it cannot. She also agreed that the health literacy of the provider is as important as that of the patient. Providers need to enhance their health literacy skills. One key is the power of observation on the provider side. It requires ongoing observation of patient understanding and perception. It is a difficult but important thing to research because it affects outcomes.

Partida reflected on the importance of maintaining a balance between health literacy research aimed at understanding the needs of and developing interventions for individual patients on the one hand and research on health system complexity needs for health literacy on the other. Health systems are driven by policy, funding, and licensing requirements. Managing such an organization while being responsive to individual patients can be a daunting task. Health literacy must be simultaneously addressed from both the patient perspective and the delivery system perspective while also recognizing diversity at each of those levels, Partida said.

Linda Harris, roundtable member at the Department of Health and Human Services (HHS), reminded the group that health literacy is an underlying theme of many of the Healthy People 2020 objectives that have to do with health communications and health information technology. The Healthy People 2020 document has been completed and is in the review and clearance process at the HHS.

Ratzan highlighted the need for increased transdisciplinary research. The idea of behavioral economics is also important, he said, and suggested that the book *Nudge* may have some lessons for health care reform (Thaler et al., 2008). There are approaches to adding behavioral incentives for everything from organ donations to choices in Medicare and Medicaid. There are clearly activities where health literacy can be integrated in CMS activities. Furthermore, health literacy is important to health care reform in many ways. These efforts can lead to better patient outcomes and public health outcomes and play into cost effective delivery of care in the 21st century, Ratzan said.

Isham closed the session by thanking all the participants for their thoughts and contributions.

References

Apter, AJ, Paasche-Orlow MK, Remillard JT, Bennett IM, Ben-Joseph EP, Batista RM, Hyde J, Rudd RE. 2008. Numeracy and communication with patients: they are counting on us. *J Gen Intern Med* 23(12):2117.

Baker DW. 2006. The meaning and measure of health literacy. *J Gen Intern Med* 21:878-883.

Baker DW, Gazmararian JA, Williams MV, Scott T, Parker RM, Green D, Ren J, Peel J. 2002. Functional health literacy and the risk of hospital admission among Medicare managed care enrollees. *Am J Pub Health* 92(8):1278-1283.

Baker DW, Wolf MS, Feinglass J, Thompson JA, Gazmararian JA, Huang J. 2007. Health literacy and mortality among elderly persons. *Arch Int Med* 167(14):1503-1509.

Bailey SC, Pandit AU, Yin S, Federman A, Davis TC, Parker RM, Wolf MS. 2009. Predictors of misunderstanding pediatric liquid medication instructions. *Fam Med* 41(10):715-721.

Bennett IM, Chen J, Soroui JS, White S. 2009. The contribution of health literacy to disparities in self-rated health status and preventive health behaviors in older adults. *Ann Fam Med* 7(3):204-211.

Berkman ND, DeWalt DA, Pignone MP, Sheridan SL, Lohr KN, Lux L, Sutton SF, Swinson T, Bonito AJ. 2004. *Literacy and Health Outcomes*. AHRQ Publication No. 04-E007-1. Rockville, MD: Agency for Healthcare Research and Quality.

Bickmore TW, Mitchell SE, Jack BW, Paasche-Orlow MK, Pfeifer LM, Odonnell J. 2010. Response to a relational agent by hospital patients with depressive symptoms. *Interact Comput* 22(4):289-298.

Chin MH, Walters AE, Cook SC, Huang ES. 2007. Interventions to reduce racial and ethnic disparities in healthcare. *Med Care Res Rev* 64(5 Suppl):7S-28S.

Cooper LA, Hill MN, Powe NR. 2002. Designing and evaluating interventions to eliminate racial and ethnic disparities in health care. *J Gen Intern Med* 17:477-486.

Czaja SJ, Charness N, Fisk AD, Hertzog C, Nair SN, Rogers WA, Sharit J. 2006. Factors predicting the use of technology: findings from the Center for Research and Education on Aging and Technology Enhancement (CREATE). *Psychol Aging* 21(2):333-352.

Czaja SJ, Sharit J, Nair SN. 2008. Usability of the Medicare health web site. *JAMA* 300(7):790-792.

DeWalt DA, Malone RM, Bryant ME, Kosnar MC, Corr KE, Rothman RL, Sueta CA, Pignone MP. 2006. A heart failure self-management program for patients of all literacy levels: a randomized, controlled trial [ISRCTN11535170]. *BMC Health Svcs Res* Mar 13;6:30.

DeWalt DA, Callahan LF, Hawk VH, Broucksou KA, Hink A, Rudd RE, Brach C. 2010. *Health Literacy Universal Precautions Toolkit.* AHRQ pub. No. 10-0046-EF. Available at: www.ahrq.gov/qual/literacy (accessed June 5, 2010).

Doak L, Doak C, Root J. 2007. *Teaching Patients with Low Literacy Skills,* 2nd edn, J. B. Lippincott, Philadelphia, PA; out of print but available at: www.hsph.harvard.edu/healthliteracy (accessed June 5, 2010).

Fang MC, Panguluri P, Machtinger EL, Schillinger D. 2009. Language, literacy, and characterization of stroke among patients taking warfarin for stroke prevention: implications for health communication. *Patient Educ Couns* 75(3):403-410.

Frohlich KL, Potvin L. 2008. Transcending the known in public health practice: the inequality paradox: the population approach and vulnerable populations. *Am J Public Health* 98(2):216-221.

Harper W, Cook S, Makloul S. 2007. Teaching medical students about health literacy: 2 Chicago initiatives, *Am J Health Behav* 31(Suppl. 1):S111-S114.

(HHS) (U.S. Department of Health and Human Services). 2006. *Healthy People 2010 Midcourse Review.* Washington, DC: U.S. Government Printing Office. http://www.healthypeople.gov/data/midcourse/html/execsummary/Goal2.htm (accessed July 11, 2010).

Howard DH, Sentell T, Gazmararian JA. 2006. Impact of health literacy on socioeconomic and racial differences in health in an elderly population. *J Gen Intern Med* 21(8):857-861.

Institute of Medicine (IOM). 2004. *Health Literacy: A Prescription to End Confusion.* Washington, DC: The National Academies Press.

Jack BW, Chett BK, Anthony D, Greenwald JL, Sanchez GM, Johnson AE, Forsythe SR, O'Donnell JK, Paasche-Orlow MK, Manasseh C, Martin S, Culpepper L. 2009. A re-engineered hospital discharge program to decrease rehospitalization: a randomized trial. *Ann Intern Med.* 150:178-187.

Jensen JD, King AJ, Davis LA, Guntzviller LM. 2010. Utilization of internet technology by low-income adults: the role of health literacy, health numeracy, and computer assistance. *J Aging Health* May 21. [Epub ahead of print].

Kaplan SH, Greenfield S. 1991. Gender differences in physician-patient communication for patients seeing the same and opposite gender physicians. *Clin Res Abstracts* 39(2):627A)

Kutner M, Greenberg E, Jin Y, Paulsen C. 2006. *The Health Literacy of America's Adults: Results from the 2003 National Assessment of Adult Literacy* (NCES 2006-483). Washington, DC: U.S. Department of Education, National Center for Education Statustics.

Lalonde M. 1974. A new perspective on the health of Canadians. http://www.hc-sc.gc.ca/hcs-sss/alt_formats/hpb-dgps/pdf/pubs/1974-lalonde/lalonde_e.pdf (accessed July 29, 2010).

Machtinger EL, Wang F, Chen LL, Rodriguez M, Wu S, Schillinger D. 2007. A visual medication schedule to improve anticoagulation control: a randomized, controlled trial. *Jt Comm J Qual Saf* 33(10):625-635.

McKinlay, JD, Potter DA, Feldman HA. 1966. Non-medical influences on medical decision-making. *Soc Sci Med* 42(5):769-776.

Morris NS, MacLean CD, Littenberg B. 2006. Literacy and health outcomes: a cross-sectional study in 1002 adults with diabetes. *BMC Fam Pract.* Aug 14;7:49.PMID: 16907968.

Office of Disease Prevention and Health Promotion (ODPHP). 2010. *National Action Plan to Improve Health Literacy.* http://www.health.gov/communication/HLActionPlan/ (accessed July 29, 2010).

Osborn CY, Paasche-Orlow MK, Davis TC, Wolf MS. 2007. Health literacy: An overlooked factor in understanding HIV health disparities. *Am J Prev Med* 33(5):374-378.

Osborn CY, Cavanaugh K, Wallston KA, White RO, Rothman RL 2009. Diabetes numeracy: an overlooked factor in understanding racial disparities in glycemic control. *Diabetes Care* 32(9):1614-1619.

Paasche-Orlow MK, Riekert KA, Bilderback A, Chanmugam A, Hill P, Rand CS, Brancati FL, Krishnan JA. 2005. Tailored education may reduce health disparities in asthma self-management. *Am J Resp Crit Care Med* 172(8):980-986.

Powers BJ, Olsen MK, Oddone EZ, Thorpe CT, Bosworth HB. 2008. Literacy and blood pressure—do healthcare systems influence this relationship? A cross-sectional study. *BMC Health Serv Res*. 2008 Oct 23;8:219.

Pronovost P, Needham D, Berenholtz S, Sinopoli D, Chu H, Cosgrove S, Sexton B, Hyzy R, Welsh R, Roth G, Bander J, Kepros J, Goeschel C. 2006 An intervention to decrease catheter-related bloodstream infections in the ICU. *N Engl J Med*. Dec 28;355(26):2725-2732.

Ratzan SC, Parker RM. 2000. Introduction. In: *National Library of Medicine Current Bibliographies in Medicine: Health Literacy*. NLM Pub. No. CBM 2000-1. Selden CR, Zorn, Ratzan SC, Parker RM, Editors. Bethesda, MD: National Institutes of Health, U.S. Department of Health and Human Services.

Richter D, Paretti MC. 2008. *Teaching Interdisciplinary Collaboration: Moving Beyond "Divide and Conquer."* Virginia Tech Engineering Communications Center Department of Engineering Education. www.ctl.calpoly.edu/.../2008_Spring_InterdisciplinaryCollaboration_Paretti.ppt (accessed July 14, 2010).

Robertson DW, Martin DK, Singer PA. 2003. Interdisciplinary research: Putting the methods under the microscope. *BMC Med Res Methodol* 3:20.

Rose G. 1992. *The Strategy of Preventive Medicine*. Oxford, England: Oxford University Press.

Roter DL. 2004. Health literacy and the patient-provider relationship, in: JG Schwartzberg, JB VanGeest, CC Wang, JA Gazmararian, RM Parker, DL Roter, RE Rudd, D Schillenger (eds) *Understanding Health Literacy: Implications for Medicine and Public Health*. Chicago, IL: AMA Press. pp. 87-100.

Roter DL, Erby LH, Larson S, Ellington L. 2007. Assessing oral literacy demand in genetic counseling dialogue: preliminary test of a conceptual framework. *Soc Sci Med* 65(7):1442-1457.

Roter DL, Erby L, Larson S, Ellington L. 2009. Oral literacy demand of prenatal genetic counseling dialogue: predictors of learning. *Patient Educ Couns* 75(3):392-397.

Rothman RL, DeWalt DA, Malone R, Bryant B, Shintani A, Crigler B, Weinberger M, Pignone M. 2004. Influence of patient literacy on the effectiveness of a primary care-based diabetes disease management program. *JAMA* 292(14):1711-1716.

Rothman RL, Housam R, Weiss H, Davis D, Gregory R, Gebretsadik T, Shintani A, Elasy TA. 2006. Patient understanding of food labels: the role of literacy and numeracy. *Am J Prev Med*. 31(5):391-398.

Rudd RE. 2007. Health literacy skills of U.S. adults. *J Health Behav* 31(Supp 1): S8-S18.

Rudd RE, Anderson JE. 2006. *The Health Literacy Environment of Hospitals and Health Centers'. Partners for Action: Making Your Healthcare Facility Literacy-Friendly.* National Center for the Study of Adult Learning and Literacy and Health and Adult Literacy and Learning Initiative, Harvard School of Public Health. http://www.ncsall.net/fileadmin/resources/teach/environ_title.pdf (accessed July 29, 2010).

Sarkar U, Karter AJ, Liu JY, Adler NE, Nguyen R, Lopez A, Schillinger D. 2010. The literacy divide: health literacy and the use of an internet-based patient portal in an integrated health system—results from the Diabetes Study of Northern California (DISTANCE). *J Health Commun* 15:183-196.

Schillinger D, Bindman A, Wang F, Stewart A, Piette J. 2004. Functional health literacy and the quality of physician-patient communication among diabetes patients. *Patient Educ Counsel*, 52(3):315-323.

Schillinger D, Barton L, Karter A, Wang F, Adler N. 2006. Does literacy mediate the relationship between education and health outcomes? A study of a low-income population with diabetes. *Pub Health Rep* 121(3):245-254.

Schillinger D, Hammer H, Wang F, Palacios J, McLean I, Tang A, Youmans S, Handley M. 2008. Seeing in 3-D: examining the reach of diabetes self-management support strategies in a public health care system. *Health Educ Behav* 35(5):664-682.

Sentell TL, Halpin HA. 2006. Importance of adult literacy in understanding health disparities. *J Gen Intern Med* 21(8):862-866.

Sharif I, Tse J. 2010. Accuracy of computer-generated, Spanish-language medicine labels. *Pediatrics* 125(5):960-965

Sudore RL, Schillinger D. 2009. Interventions to improve care for patients with limited health literacy. *J Clin Outcomes Manag* 16(1):20-29.

Thaler RH, Sunstein CR. 2008. *Nudge: Improving Decisions About Health, Wealth, and Happiness.* New Haven, CT: Yale University Press.

Varkey AB, Manwell LB, Williams ES, Ibrahim SA, Brown RL, Bobula JA, Horner-Ibler BA, Schwartz MD, Konrad TR, Wiltshire JC, Linzer M; MEMO Investigators. 2009. Separate and unequal: clinics where minority and nonminority patients receive primary care. *Arch Inern Med* 169(3):243-250.

Volandes AE, Paasche-Orlow MK, Gillick MR, Cook EF, Shaykevich S, Abbo ED, Lehmann L. 2008. Health literacy not race predicts end-of-life care preferences. *J Palliat Med* 11(5):754-762.

Wolf MS, Knight SJ, Lyons EA, Durazo-Arvizu R, Pickard SA, Arseven A, Arozullah A, Colella K, Ray P, Bennett CL. 2006. Literacy, race, and PSA level among low-income men newly diagnosed with prostate cancer. *Urology* 68(1):89-93.

Yin SH, Johnson M, Mendelsohn AL, Abrams MA, Sanders LM, Dreyer BP. 2009. The health literacy of parents in the United States: a nationally representative study. *Pediatrics* 124(Suppl 3):S289-S298.

Zarcadoolas C, Pleasant A, Greer DS. 2005. Understanding health literacy: an expanded model. *Health Promo Internat* 20(2):195-203.

Appendix A

Workshop Agenda

Innovations in Health Literacy Research: A Workshop
May 27, 2010

Barbara Jordan Conference Center
Kaiser Family Foundation Building
1330 G Street, NW
Washington, DC

Thursday, May 27, 2010 **OPEN SESSION**

9:00-9:15 Welcome and Introduction to the Agenda
George Isham, M.D., M.S.
Chair, IOM Roundtable on Health Literacy
Medical Director and Chief Health Officer
HealthPartners

9:15-9:45 Presentation of Report on the First Annual Research on Health Literacy Conference
Michael Paasche-Orlow, M.D., M.A., M.P.H.
Associate Professor of Medicine
Boston University School of Medicine

9:45-10:45 The Role of Health Literacy in Health Disparities Research
Suggested Speakers:

9:45-10:00 How do we raise awareness of health literacy among disparity researchers? How can we keep research in disparities and research in health literacy from being in separate silos?
Lisa Cooper, M.D., M.P.H.
Professor, Health Policy & Management & Health, Behavior, and Society
Johns Hopkins Bloomberg School of Public Health

10:00-10:15 How can health literacy help eliminate disparities? How does health literacy impact vulnerable populations?
Dean Schillinger, M.D.
Professor of Clinical Medicine
University of California, San Francisco

10:15-10:45 Discussion

10:45-11:00 BREAK

11:00-12:00 The Role of Health Literacy in Health Information Technology

11:00-11:15 How do we make sure health IT does not leave individuals with limited health literacy in the dust? What kind of research is needed to look at this issue?
Joshua Seidman, Ph.D.
Acting Director, Meaningful Use
Office of Provider Adoption Support
Office of the National Coordinator for Health Information Technology

11:15-11:30 How do we use health IT to help those with limited health literacy: potentials, concerns, how do we study this?
Michael Wolf, Ph.D., M.P.H.
Associate Professor, Medicine and Learning Sciences
Associate Division Chief - Research
Division of General Internal Medicine
Feinberg School of Medicine
Northwestern University

11:30-12:00 Discussion

12:00-1:00 LUNCH

1:00-2:00 Professional Development in Health Literacy Research: How Do We Build the Field of Health Literacy Research?

1:00-1:15 ***David Baker, M.D., M.P.H.***
Professor, Department of Medicine
Chief, General Internal Medicine
Feinberg School of Medicine
Northwestern University

1:15-1:30 ***Debra Roter, Dr. P.H.***
Professor
Johns Hopkins Bloomberg School of Public Health

1:30-2:00 Discussion

2:00-2:30 National Action Plan to Improve Health Literacy

Cynthia Baur, Ph.D.
Senior Advisor, Health Literacy
Centers for Disease Control and Prevention

Raynard Kington, M.D., Ph.D.
Deputy Director
National Institutes of Health

Carolyn Clancy, M.D.
Director
Agency for Healthcare Research and Quality
U.S. Department of Health and Human Services

2:30-3:00 Discussion

3:00-3:45 The Role of Health Literacy Research in the National Action Plan
Suggested Speakers:

3:00-3:15 ***Terry C. Davis, Ph.D.***
Professor
Departments of Medicine and Pediatrics
Louisiana State University Health Sciences Center

3:15-3:30 ***Rima Rudd, Sc.D.***
Senior Lecturer on Society, Human Development & Health
Director of Educational Programs
Department of Society, Human Development and Health
Harvard School of Public Health

3:30-4:00 Discussion

4:00-4:15 Summary of Lessons Learned from Workshop
George Isham

Appendix B

Workshop Speaker Biosketches

David W. Baker, M.D., M.P.H., is the Michael A. Gertz Professor of Medicine, Chief of the Division of General Internal Medicine, and Director of the REACH Practice-Based Research Network at the Feinberg School of Medicine, Northwestern University in Chicago. Dr. Baker's research activities have focused on health care delivery for underserved populations and improving quality of care for chronic medical conditions. He was one of the Principal Investigators for the Literacy in Health Care Study, the first major study examining how often patients are unable to accurately read pill bottles, appointment slips, and the other written materials they encounter when they come to see a doctor. He was also the Principal Investigator for a large study of literacy, health status, use of health care services, and mortality that included over 3000 Medicare managed care enrollees in 4 cities in the U.S. He was one of the developers of the Test of Functional Health Literacy in Adults, and he has published extensively on the measurement of health literacy and the consequences of inadequate health literacy. His current work focuses on developing interventions to improve health communication and to improve patient self-management skills and health behaviors, including use of multimedia and health information technology. He also leads several projects examining the use of electronic health record systems for clinical decision support, quality improvement, and rapid dissemination of new medical advances.

Cynthia Baur, Ph.D., is the Senior Advisor for Health Literacy, Office of the Associate Director for Communication, Centers for Disease Control and Prevention (CDC), U.S. Department of Health and Human Services (HHS). From 2006–2010, she was the Director, Division of Health Communication and Marketing, National Center for Health Marketing, CDC. She is a cochair of the Healthy People 2020 Health Communication and Health Information Technology Workgroup and a cochair of the HHS workgroup on health literacy. She is the lead author of the National Action Plan to Improve Health Literacy and one of the developers of CDC's online health literacy training for health professionals. Dr. Baur holds a Ph.D. in Communication from the University of California, San Diego.

Carolyn M. Clancy, M.D., was appointed Director of the Agency for Healthcare Research and Quality (AHRQ) on February 5, 2003 and reappointed on October 9, 2009. Prior to her appointment, Dr. Clancy was Director of AHRQ's Center for Outcomes and Effectiveness Research.

Dr. Clancy, a general internist and health services researcher, is a graduate of Boston College and the University of Massachusetts Medical School. Following clinical training in internal medicine, Dr. Clancy was a Henry J. Kaiser Family Foundation Fellow at the University of Pennsylvania. Before joining AHRQ in 1990, she was also an assistant professor in the Department of Internal Medicine at the Medical College of Virginia.

Dr. Clancy holds an academic appointment at George Washington University School of Medicine (Clinical Associate Professor, Department of Medicine) and serves as Senior Associate Editor, Health Services Research. She serves on multiple editorial boards including the Annals of Internal Medicine, Annals of Family Medicine, American Journal of Medical Quality, and Medical Care Research and Review.

She is a member of the Institute of Medicine and was elected a Master of the American College of Physicians in 2004. In 2009, was awarded the 2009 William B. Graham Prize for Health Services Research.

Her major research interests include improving health care quality and patient safety, and reducing disparities in care associated with patients' race, ethnicity, gender, income, and education. As Director, she launched the first annual report to the Congress on health care disparities and health care quality.

Lisa Cooper, M.D., M.P.H., is Professor of Health Policy & Management, and Health Behavior & Society at the Johns Hopkins Bloomberg School of Public Health. Dr. Cooper's research program focuses on patient-centered strategies for improving outcomes and overcoming racial and ethnic disparities in healthcare. She has conducted several observational studies to explore and better define barriers (e.g., patient attitudes, beliefs, and preferences) to equitable care across racial and ethnic groups and mechanisms for disparities in health status and healthcare (e.g., patient-physician communication, race discordance between patients and physicians, physicians' implicit attitudes about race). Dr. Cooper was the principal investigator of two randomized trials funded by the National Heart, Lung, and Blood Institute (NHLBI) and the Agency for Healthcare Research and Quality (AHRQ) of interventions to improve quality of care and outcomes for patients with hypertension and depression in primary care settings. She also has a Mid-Career Investigator Award for Patient-Oriented Research in Cardiovascular Health Disparities from the NHLBI and she is the principal investigator of a new NHLBI-funded Center for Population Health and Health Disparities. Dr. Cooper has been an elected IOM member since 2008.

Dr. Cooper's research links patient and clinician attitudes and behaviors with health outcomes; her work continues to inform the training of physicians and the institutions in which they practice to deliver high quality, equitable care to increasingly diverse patient populations.

Terry C. Davis, Ph.D., is a Professor of Medicine and Pediatrics at Louisiana State University Health Sciences Center in Shreveport where she also heads the Behavioral Science unit at the Feist-Weiller Cancer Center. For the past 25 years, she has led an interdisciplinary team investigating the impact of patient literacy on health and healthcare. Seminal achievements include development of the Rapid Estimate of Adult Literacy in Medicine (REALM) and creation of user- friendly patient education and provider training materials.

Dr. Davis has more than one hundred publications related to health literacy, health communication and preventive medicine. She has served on Health Literacy Advisory Boards for both the American Medical Association and the American College of Physicians Foundation (ACP-F). Dr. Davis was an independent agent on the IOM Committee on Health Literacy and a developer of the AMA's Train-the-Trainer Health Literacy Curriculum. Currently she is a member of the Healthy People 2010 Health Literacy/Health Communication Section and serves on the FDA's Drug Safety and Risk Management Advisory Committee.

Dr. Davis is Principal Investigator on a 5 year NCI health literacy intervention to increase regular breast and CRC screening among patients in Federally Qualified Health Centers. She is also working with investigators at Northwestern, Emory and Harvard on AHRQ funded studies to improve patient understanding of prescription medication labels in English and Spanish. Along with a team from the University of North Carolina, University of California San Francisco and Northwestern she has been funded by the ACP-F to develop and test practical self-management guides and videos for patients with diabetes, COPD, and coronary artery disease. The ACP-F has distributed more than a million copies of these guides and videos. She is also a coinvestigator on a CDC funded project to teach vaccine safety through the Academic Pediatric Association's on line curriculum for residents and practicing physicians.

Raynard Kington, M.D., Ph.D., is the Principal Deputy Director of the National Institutes of Health (NIH). Dr. Kington has held this position since February 9, 2003. He served as Acting NIH Director from October 31, 2008 until the appointment of Dr. Francis S. Collins on August 17, 2009. During his tenure as Acting NIH Director, he led the agency through the development of NIH's plan for the use of the $10.4 billion American Recovery and Reinvestment Act resources designed to accelerate biomedical science and the economy. In July, 2009, NIH published the final "NIH Guidelines for Human Stem Cell Research" under his directorship. With the appointment of the current director, Dr. Francis S. Collins (August 17, 2009), Kington resumed his role as Principal Deputy Director. Prior to his present appointment, Dr. Kington was Director of the Office of Behavioral and Social Sciences Research (2000-2003). In addition to this role, from January, 2002 to November, 2002, he served as Acting Director of the National Institute on Alcohol Abuse and Alcoholism.

Before coming to NIH, Dr. Kington was Director of the Division of Health Examination Statistics at the National Center for Health Statistics (NCHS) of the Centers for Disease Control and Prevention (CDC). As Division Director, he also served as Director of the National Health and Nutrition Examination Survey (NHANES), one of the nation's largest studies to assess the health of the American people. Prior to coming to NCHS, he was a Senior Scientist in the Health Program at the RAND Corporation. While at RAND, Dr. Kington was a Co-Director of the Drew/RAND Center on Health and Aging, a National Institute on Aging Exploratory Minority Aging Center.

Dr. Kington attended the University of Michigan, where he received his B.S. with distinction and his M.D. He subsequently completed his residency in Internal Medicine at Michael Reese Medical Center in Chicago. He was then appointed a Robert Wood Johnson Clinical Scholar at the University of Pennsylvania. While at the University of Pennsylvania, he completed his M.B.A. with distinction and his Ph.D. with a concentration in Health Policy and Economics at the Wharton School and was awarded a Fontaine Fellowship. He is board-certified in Internal Medicine and Public Health and Preventive Medicine. In 2006, Dr. Kington was elected to membership in the Institute of Medicine of the National Academy of Sciences.

Dr. Kington's research has focused on the role of social factors, especially socioeconomic status, as determinants of health. His research has included studies of the health and socioeconomic status of black immigrants, demographic correlates of the willingness to participate in genetic research, the relationship between wealth and health status, the health status of U.S. Hispanic populations, and the determinants of health care services utilization.

Michael Paasche-Orlow, M.D., M.A., M.P.H., Associate Professor of Medicine, Boston University School of Medicine, is a nationally recognized expert in health literacy. Dr. Paasche-Orlow's work has focused on patient-centered interventions that utilize health information technologies that are accessible for people with limited literacy and is currently a co-investigator for seven funded studies. Dr. Paasche-Orlow is the Associate Director of the Boston University School of Medicine, General Internal Medicine Fellowship Program and is currently mentoring 6 fellows and junior faculty members. He conducted his own postdoctoral research in clinical epidemiology, health services research, and bioethics in the Division of General Internal Medicine, Johns Hopkins School of Medicine. Prior to that, he completed his residency training in the Primary Care track of the NYU-Bellevue Internal Medicine training program and medical school at the Albert Einstein School of Medicine.

Debra Roter, Dr.P.H., is Professor of Health, Behavior and Society at the Johns Hopkins Bloomberg School of Public Health and holds appointments of Professor in the Schools of Medicine and Nursing and with the Kimmel Comprehensive Cancer Center.

Dr. Roter's primary research focus is in the study of patient-health care provider communication. She is the author of the Roter Interaction Analysis System (RIAS), a method of process analysis applied to medical exchange widely used by researchers and educators nationally and internationally. Her studies include basic social psychology research regarding social and psychological determinants and consequences of interpersonal influence within medical encounters, patient and provider interventions to improve health care quality, and communication and educational applications to enhance patient and provider communication skills.

Dr. Roter has authored over 200 articles and book chapters and three books related to the subject of patient-health care provider communication. She is recognized by the Web of Science as among highly cited authors in the social sciences.

Dr. Roter is currently Principal Investigator of an NICHD funded study to assess oral literacy burden of medical communication and to develop an ameliorative patient activation intervention for pregnant women with poor literacy skills.

Rima Rudd, Sc.D., is the Senior Lecturer on Society, Human Development, and Health at the Harvard School of Public Health. Her work centers on health communication and on the design and evaluation of public health community based programs. She has been teaching courses on innovative strategies in health education, program planning and evaluation, psychosocial and behavioral theory, and health literacy since 1988.

Dr. Rudd is focusing her research inquiries on literacy related disparities and literacy related barriers to health programs, services, and care, working closely with the adult education, public health, oral health, and medical sectors.

Dr. Rudd wrote several reports that help shape the agenda in health literacy research and practice. They include the health literacy chapter of the Health and Human Services report Communicating Health: Priorities and Strategies for Progress (2003), the Educational Testing Services report, Literacy and Health in America (2004), and two in-depth literature reviews (Review of Adult Learning and Literacy volume 1 in 2000 and volume 7 in 2007). She served on the Institute of Medicine Committee on Health Literacy, the National Research Council Committee on Measuring Adult Literacy, the National Institute of Dental and Craniofacial Research Workgroup on Oral Health Literacy, on the Joint Commission Advisory Committee on Health Literacy and Patient Safety and contributed to the ensuing reports and white papers.

Dr. Rudd currently serves on the National Health Literacy Advisory Board for the American Dental Association and is the Senior Health Literacy Advisor for the Missouri Foundation. She is a visiting professor in the Faculty of Health and Social Care, London Southbank University and is appointed the visiting Health Literacy Scholar at the Horowitz Center on Health Literacy at the University of Maryland, School of Public Health. She is a coprincipal investigator on several ongoing health literacy research projects. Rima Rudd is considered a leader in this growing field of research and practice.

Dean Schillinger, M.D., is Professor of Medicine in Residence at the University of California, San Francisco, and Acting Chief of the UCSF Division of General Internal Medicine at San Francisco General Hospital (SFGH). He is also a practicing primary care physician at SFGH, an urban public hospital, where he sees patients, teaches in the primary care residency program, and conducts research. He is the Director of the UCSF Center for Vulnerable Populations, a new research center committed to transforming clinical and public health practice by improving health communication for socially vulnerable people, and is a member of a UCSF-wide translational research committee to expand the scope and quality of implementation and dissemination sciences.

Dr. Schillinger also serves as Chief of the Diabetes Prevention and Control Program for the California Department of Public Health, where he has been expanding the program's work in health communications, social and environmental determinants of diabetes, and health disparities. In his prior administrative roles, he has directed the Medi-Cal managed care clinic at SFGH, the ambulatory care clinics at SFGH, and has been the Director of Clinical Operations for the Department of Medicine.

Author of over 100 scientific manuscripts, Dr. Schillinger carries out research related to healthcare for vulnerable populations, and focuses on literacy, health communication, and chronic disease prevention and management. He has carried out a number of studies exploring the impact of limited health literacy on the care of patients with diabetes and heart disease. He has been honored with the 2003 Institute for Healthcare Advancement Research Award; the 2008 Research Award in Safety and Quality from the National Patient Safety Foundation; the 2009 Engel Award in Health Communication Research; and the California Association of Public Hospital Quality Leaders Award for this work. He has been the recipient of grants from NIH, The California Endowment, The Commonwealth Fund, AHRQ, and the California Health Care Foundation to develop and evaluate care management programs tailored to the literacy and language needs of patients with chronic disease, and was a cofounder for the National Association of Public Health and Hospital Institute's Diabetes Quality Improvement Consortium.

Dr. Schillinger contributed to the 2004 Institute of Medicine Report on Health Literacy, is a section editor for the textbooks Understanding Health Literacy (AMA press) and Caring for Vulnerable and Underserved Populations (Lange series, 2007), and is a member of the American College of Physician's Health Communication Advisory Board, and serves on the Editorial Board of the journal Patient Education and Counseling. He completed an Open Society Institute Advocacy Fellowship working with California Literacy, Inc., a nonprofit educational organization that helps people gain literacy skills, to advance the California Health Literacy Initiative. With respect to chronic disease control on the global level, he recently returned from a semester as Visiting Scholar at the University of Chile's School of Public Health to help develop chronic disease prevention and treatment initiatives, has served as a consultant to the National Health Group in Singapore on its chronic disease and health promotion initiatives.

Joshua Seidman, Ph.D., at ONC, guides development of tools and resources that help providers become meaningful users of HIT, and helps to evolve meaningful use practice and policy. During nearly two decades in health care, Seidman has focused on quality measurement and improvement; the intersection of e-health and health services research; and structuring consumer e-health interventions to support improved health behaviors and informed decision making. Previously, Seidman founded the Center for Information Therapy, which advanced the practice and science of delivering tailored information to consumers to help them make better health decisions and lead healthier lives. At the IxCenter, Seidman focused on stimulating innovation, diffusing best practices, and evangelizing for a patient centered orientation to implementation of HIT applications. Dr. Seidman has a PhD in health services research and an MHS in health policy and management from the Johns Hopkins School of Public Health, and a BA in political science from Brown University.

Michael S. Wolf, Ph.D., M.P.H., is an associate professor of medicine, associate division chief of research, and director of the Center for Communication in Healthcare at the Feinberg School of Medicine at Northwestern University. Dr. Wolf is a behavioral scientist and health services researcher with primary interests in adult literacy and learning, cognitive factors, and the management of chronic disease. He was one of the first recipients of the Pfizer Health Literacy Initiative Scholar Award and has received numerous national awards for his work in the field of health literacy and medication safety.

Dr. Wolf has written 84 peer-reviewed publications, many of which address the problem of limited health literacy. He currently serves on advisory committees for the U.S. Food and Drug Administration, U.S. Pharmacopeia, the American Dental Association, and the Agency for Healthcare Research and Quality. He has repeatedly provided consultation to the Institute of Medicine, American College of Physicians Foundation, American Medical Association, American Pharmacists Association, and Centers for Disease Control on health literacy matters.

He is the principal investigator on grants from the National Institute on Aging, National Cancer Institute, Agency for Healthcare Research and Quality, Target Corporation, Foundation for Informed Decision Making, and the Missouri Foundation for Health. Dr. Wolf also led an Institute of Medicine white paper on health literacy and medication safety, and he is the principal investigator of a trial to test enhanced drug labeling and the use of visual aids to improve patient processing and understanding of medication instructions.

Appendix C

Workshop Report from the Health Literacy Annual Research Conference

Conference Date: October 19–20, 2009

Presented by Michael Paasche-Orlow, M.D., M.A., M.P.H.
Boston University School of Medicine, Department of Medicine, Section of General Internal Medicine, Boston, Massachusetts

The Health Literacy Annual Research Conference (HARC) is an interdisciplinary meeting for investigators dedicated to health literacy research. Our aim is to attract a full range of investigators engaged in health literacy research including those involved in a broad array of public health, health services, epidemiology, translational, and interventional research activities.

The first HARC took place in October 2009 at the National Academy of Sciences Building. This meeting was coordinated with the assistance of Rose Martinez on behalf of the Institute of Medicine Roundtable on Health Literacy and sponsored by a grant from the National Center on Minority Health and Health Disparities (NCMHD), Project Officer - Robert Netty, with additional significant support from the Agency for Healthcare Research and Quality (AHRQ), Project Officer - Cindy Brach. Additional coordination and support was provided by Helen Meissner, of the Office of Behavioral and Social Sciences Research (OBSSR) as well as the National Institute of Biomedical Imaging & Bioengineering (NIBIB), Project Officer - John Haller and the Eunice Kennedy Shriver National Institute of Child Health and Human Development (NICHD), Project Officer - Lynne Haverkos. Principal Investigator Michael Paasche-Orlow, MD, MPH, 1 R13 MD003392.

--*-*-*

A second year of funding from the National Center on Minority Health and Health Disparities (NCMHD), Project Officer - Robert Netty, with additional significant support from the Agency for Healthcare Research and Quality (AHRQ), Project Officer - Cindy Brach, has been secured.

HARC II will take place October 18–19, 2010, at the Hyatt Regency, Bethesda, MD. For more information please visit the HARC II website: http://www.bumc.bu.edu/healthliteracyconference/.

It will be an opportunity to advance the field of health literacy, a method to raise the quality of our research, and a venue for professional development.

Table of Contents

I. Executive Summary

The HARC conference took place over 2 full days in October 2009 and highlighted areas of important research advancement as well as important lacunae in the field. A keynote address by David Baker, MD, MPH examined the role health literacy in patient education and a keynote address by Anne Beal, MD, MPH, focused on the role of health literacy in health disparities. There were four panels of invited speakers dealing with (1) measurement; (2) health literacy and verbal interactions; (3) health information technology interventions; and (4) organizational assessment and change. Current gaps in the research were examined by invited speakers and in breakout sessions relating to Public Health Approaches to Health Literacy, Health Disparities and Health Literacy, and Health Information Technology. An additional 62 posters and 12 oral abstracts were presented, making this clearly the most numerous Health Literacy research presentations in any single meeting to date. The meeting was attended by an interdisciplinary array of investigators representing the strong majority of health literacy investigators in the United States.

This report describes the rationale for having a Health Literacy Annual Research Conference, the goals for the meeting, and presents the findings of the meeting. In addition, specific discussion is presented regarding two of the recurring themes of the meeting, namely, the Role of Health Literacy Research in Health Disparities and the Role of Information Technology in Health Literacy Research.

Details from the 2009 conference, including panel presentations, accepted abstracts, and evaluation results, can be found on the conference website at http://www.bumc.bu.edu/healthliteracyconference/2009-conference/.

II. Why the Health Literacy Annual Research Conference (HARC) Was Initiated

Introduction

The National Institutes of Health (NIH) has defined health literacy as the "degree to which individuals have the capacity to obtain, process and understand basic health information and services needed to make appropriate health decisions."[1] According to this definition, health literacy relates to an individual's possession of requisite skills for making health-related decisions. As highlighted in the IOM report, health literacy is dependent on the complexity of the tasks required.[2] This means that when we refer to health literacy, we consider not only a patient's literacy and numeracy skills, but also the literacy burden imposed by health care systems and communities in which care-giving and self-management support take place.[3,4]

Unfortunately, many of the tasks health consumers need to undertake are very complicated. Over the past 50 years, basic literacy has improved in the United States. However, over 90 million American adults struggle to read and understand basic health materials.[5] Thus, given the high literacy demands required to function successfully as a patient, it is no wonder that approximately 36% of US adults have only basic or even below basic health literacy skills.[6] This problem is not uniformly distributed in society; the prevalence of limited health literacy is highest among patients who are older and are from ethnic and racial minorities.[7]

The literature on health literacy also exposes ways in which the health care system exacerbates the impact of underlying educational and income disparities. Indeed, health literacy is emerging as an important causal factor for racial and ethnic health disparities.[8-18] The implications of this research should be understood as a challenge to the basic justice of a health care system organized for the most highly educated and powerful members of our society.[19]

The relationship between limited literacy and adverse health outcomes has been well documented, and seminal reports about the problem of limited health literacy have been issued by the Institute of Medicine, [20] Agency for Healthcare Research and Quality, [21] American Medical Association, [22] and Joint Commission on the Accreditation of Hospital Organizations[23] among others. Each of these reports advocates further research to develop an effective response within health care systems to address the problem and research in health literacy has begun to flourish.

An important next step for cultivating this emerging research field is to create a national professional interdisciplinary home for investigators dedicated to health literacy research. Opportunities are available, but only within special interest groups that have either formed in more specialized meetings or that sporadically address health literacy (e.g., National Society of General Internal Medicine Annual Meeting, National American Public Health Association Annual Meeting, Academy Health, and the International Conference on Communication in Health Care). There are, in addition, multiple Health Literacy meetings (e.g., the Annual Institute for Healthcare Advancement Conference) which serve primarily an educational agenda for attendees who are, by and large, not health literacy investigators.

Timeliness

A Pubmed search using the Health Literacy topic specific query under the Pubmed tools tab (see: http://www.nlm.nih.gov/services/health_literacy.html) reveals the tremendous growth of research in this field: in the 5 years between 1986 and 1990 there are 129 references in Pubmed; in the years 1991 to 1995 this search yields 306 references; between 1996 and 2000 there are 307 references; from 2001 to 2005 there are 602 references from this search; and in the current interval, between 2006 and 6/6/2010, there are already 1,576 references returned by this search (see Figure). As striking as this may seem, it is also important to note that this collection of references is dominated by observational research, indeed, fewer than 8% of these citations are tagged as trials as seen in the figure below.

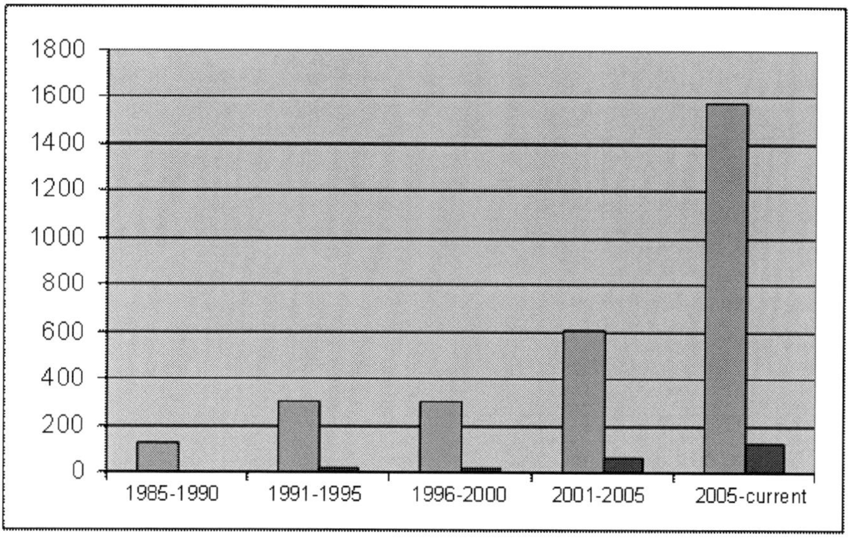

Light bars represent all citations identified by Health Literacy topic specific query. Dark bars represent the subset of these citations identified as trials, clinical trials, or randomized controlled trials.

Despite the rapid growth in the field, driven in large part by the availability of NIH and AHRQ funding, there is currently no national research venue dedicated to the promotion of health literacy as a field of inquiry. Health literacy research is an interdisciplinary endeavor and could greatly benefit at this point from a recurring national research oriented interdisciplinary meeting.

III. Main Conference Goals

Establishing an interdisciplinary research home for health literacy investigators would be useful for reasons that relate to (1) professional development, (2) advancing the science of health literacy research, and (3) promotion of interdisciplinary research.

1. Professional Development:

Such a venue could help attract young investigators and new ideas and methods to the field. An annual meeting could be a source and meeting place for mentoring and be an opportunity to establish and advance a career in the field of health literacy. The budget and meeting schedule reflect these priorities by setting aside money to support young investigators and students and by dedicating time at the meeting for one-on-one mentoring sessions and meetings with program officers.

2. Advancing the Science:

An annual meeting of health literacy researchers could promote the discourse in this field of inquiry. For example, significant controversy exists within the field regarding core definitional issues. This is having a big influence in the arena of measurement. There is broad agreement that current health literacy instruments are insufficient in various ways for many investigators. Investigators have been developing and evaluating new instruments that reflect their understanding of what is or is not part of the concept health literacy. The proposed conferences will allow investigators to more fully debate these issues, more rapidly vet emerging measurement ideas, share early-stage instruments to allow validation activities in various populations, and disseminate newly validated instruments.

3. Promotion of Interdisciplinary Research:

Establishing a collegial network could help promote multisite research. The field has entered into an exciting and creative period of inquiry in which a wide array of interventions is being evaluated. The varied nature of the research that is relevant to the problem of health literacy makes an interdisciplinary conference valuable; bringing such a group of researchers together will provide the milieu for new admixtures, new collaborations, and further creativity. Productive collaboration will also support professional development of the health literacy investigator workforce.

Currently, the majority of health literacy research is conducted in the United States. However, health literacy research is being pursued in other countries. In 2009, Drs. Paasche-Orlow and Wolf served as guest editors for a special issue on health literacy of the journal Patient Education and Counseling. In this capacity, they have been in contact with researchers engaged in health literacy work in England, Germany, Australia, Canada, Netherlands, Israel, France, Korea, and Japan. We are aware of differences in how the field of health literacy is evolving in different parts of the world and plan to have this conference be a meeting place in which international communication and collaboration can be fostered.

Conference Proceedings

The conference took place over 2 full days in October 2009 (see Section VI for the detailed agenda). The sessions included (1) keynote addresses by David Baker, MD, MPH and Anne Beal, MD, MPH, (2) invited panels on measurement, health literacy and verbal interactions, health information technology interventions, and organizational assessment and change, and (3) oral abstract sessions which included presentations of the highest rated abstracts submitted to the conference. In total, 96 abstracts were submitted for review and 74 were accepted for presentation in either poster (62) or oral (12) form.

The panel and abstract presentations are available on our conference website at http://www.bumc.bu.edu/healthliteracyconference/2009-conference/.

In addition, on the first morning of the conference, Helen Meissner, PhD, Senior Advisor, OBSSR, coordinated a session titled NIH Gaps and Priorities for Future Research. The session was moderated by Ruth Parker, MD. The overall purpose of this session was to identify remaining gaps in our current understanding of the problems that underlie health literacy and approaches to address them. Program officers at the NIH, AHRQ, and CDC, were interested in soliciting investigator input regarding research gaps in the field.

Prior to the conference, registrants were invited to submit ideas regarding broad categories of gaps in our understanding of health literacy. We then invited speakers to address some of the major gaps in a plenary session, after which we broke into smaller groups for further discussion. The major gap topics were

- Public Health Approaches to Health Literacy
- Health Disparities and Health Literacy
- Health Information Technology

See the conference website at http://www.bumc.bu.edu/healthliteracyconference/2009-conference/ for a list of speakers and summary of the themes gleaned from these sessions.

Attendance, Evaluation Summary, and Dissemination

The First Annual HARC was very well attended. An online registration site was created, and 206 people registered for the conference, and 198 attended. Participants included the strong majority of all active health literacy researchers in the United States. Two principle dissemination activities were arranged: (1) the Institute of Medicine: Health Literacy Roundtable Workshop on the findings of the HARC meeting, and (2) a special issue on Health Literacy from presentations of the HARC meeting of the Journal of Health Communication. The guest editors of the special issue are Michael Paasche-Orlow, Lauren McCormack, and Elizabeth Wilson. The special issue will be published in September 2010. See the conference website at http://www.bumc.bu.edu/healthliteracyconference/2009-conference/ for complete results of the evaluation.

IV. Theme 1—Role of Health Literacy Research in Health Disparities Research

In the United States, racial/ethnic and socioeconomic disparities within the educational system have long been reported. As a result, two thirds of African American adults and 74% of Hispanic adults have limited functional literacy skills, compared to 32% of whites.[24] The consequences of early failures in education have more recently been linked to problems in healthcare. More than half (58%) of African American adults and 66% of Hispanic adults have limited "health literacy" skills, while less than a third of whites face such problems.[25] Research has begun to emerge showing how a health literacy skill set is linked to a range of health outcomes, and evidence has also emerged demonstrating how deficits in these skills possibly explain certain disparities.

As one of the primary public health goals in the U.S. and other industrialized countries is to better understand and respond to health disparities, a health literacy perspective provides an important new direction for seeking perhaps more potentially modifiable strategies for reducing inequities in the short-term, with a multitude of targets. Health literacy researchers are now recognizing the need for comprehensive strategies that go beyond considering only a patient's functional literacy abilities. Rather, health literacy interventions should examine the complexity of the tasks required of patients and families within healthcare settings, the accessibility of providers for the target populations, the preparedness of health and public health professionals to engage productively with patients, and the features of the health care system, working environments, and communities in which caregiving and self-management support take place.

Health literacy research calls attention to the ways in which unnecessarily complex healthcare exacerbates the impact of underlying educational and income disparities. The implications of this extensive body of literature should be understood as a direct challenge to health systems that have been organized for the most highly educated and affluent members of a society. While seminal reports about the problem of limited health literacy have been issued by the Institute of Medicine, [20] Agency for Healthcare Research and Quality, [21] American Medical Association, [22] and Joint Commission on the Accreditation of Hospital Organizations[23] among others, none have focused on how health literacy research may help eliminate disparities.

Opportunities to integrate these fields of inquiry are likely to be mutually beneficial. Yet, currently health literacy and health disparities research typically occur in their own silos. Several key aspects of how research in health literacy can help eliminate health disparities are discussed.

A. Integrate Health Literacy Assessment in Disparities Research

The first step in measurement. Without measurement, it is not possible to know when and how health literacy may be relevant to various forms of disparities, and it would be very easy to design interventions that fail to attend to relevant factors. For example, in an adjusted analysis that excluded literacy, African Americans were 2.40 times more likely to be non-adherent to their HIV-medication regimen than whites (95% confidence interval [CI]=1.14–5.08). When literacy was included in the final model adjusting for relevant covariates, the effect estimates of race diminished to non-significance and health literacy remained a significant independent predictor of non-adherence (adjusted odds ratio [AOR]=2.12, 95% CI=1.93–2.32).[26] In another study, patients were asked their preferences regarding end-of-life care after hearing a verbal description of advanced dementia and then they were asked to relay their preferences again after viewing a 2 minute video of a patient with advanced dementia. The African American subjects were found to prefer more aggressive care than the white subjects. When health literacy was included in the final model, health literacy—but not race—was significant and independent predictor of preferences for care (low literacy OR 7.1, 95% CI 2.1–24.2; marginal literacy 5.1, 95% CI 1.6–16.3).[27] Health literacy clearly mediated the influence of race on end-of-life preferences. In both of these investigations, completely different conclusions would have been made without concurrent evaluation of race and health literacy.

B. Improve Patient Education

Patients at every education level will benefit from a reduction of paperwork, plain and simple communication, and standardized processes. Satisfaction, comprehension, and retention of information are enhanced for all patients when they are presented with plain language materials.[28] While a fair amount of research has already focused on methods of patient education, there is still a tremendous unfulfilled agenda. There remain many open questions about approaches to optimizing the types of simplification called for by the health literacy literature and the types of cultural tailoring called for by the cultural competence literature.

C. Simplification of the health care system: Access and Utilization

Unneeded complexity in healthcare exacerbates the impact of underlying educational disparities. The healthcare system is not the cause of the educational disparities that exist in the US; however, without simplification in all arenas (access, patient-clinician interactions, support of self-care) the health care system transforms educational disparities into health disparities. Benefit systems need to be designed to succeed. Complex application forms, terms, and documentation requirements are significant barriers that disproportionately burden vulnerable populations.[29-30] A health literacy lens should be taken to all public programs: How will a person with limited literacy get and use this program?

D. Simplification of the health care system: Education and Training of Health Professionals

Health professionals contribute to the unneeded complexity of the healthcare system with poor communication and limited dedication to patient education. Clinicians frequently use jargon,[31] rarely confirm if their patients understand what is being discussed,[32] and patients frequently misunderstand a broad array of critical information.[33] Health literacy curricula need to be integrated into professional education and such efforts need to be evaluated. To date, there is a dearth of research on the impact of educational initiatives to promote the knowledge and skills of health professionals regarding health literacy. Curricular initiatives to address health disparities are further advanced. There is a National Consortium for Multicultural Education for Health Professionals including educators from 18 US medical schools, which collect lessons learned from curriculum implementation to guide similar educational endeavors across the consortium.[34] Indeed, several states have laws and or regulations that mandate training health professions in cultural competence (https://www.thinkculturalhealth.org/cc_legislation.asp). Inclusion of health literacy in such policy initiatives can help promulgate health literacy curricula, but research will be needed to identify programs that work, can be replicated, and help eliminate health disparities.

E. Simplification of the health care system: Self-Care

High-quality medical care integrates evidence-based clinical care with a patient-centered orientation. A patient-centered orientation for health care is one that (1) includes pre-activation to prepare patients and tailor appropriate messages; (2) prioritizes collaborative goal-setting and relationship-centered care during the visit; (3) delivers post visit reinforcements and follow-up services for both cognitive and behavioral outcomes; (4) offers proactive surveillance during the inter-visit period to identify unanticipated changes in health trajectory or access difficulties; and (5) broadens the array of available self-management support strategies. The systematic delivery of these steps requires more than a motivated clinician; it requires a redesigned medical home as described by the Care Model. A growing body of literature suggests that tailored implementation of elements of the Care Model can disproportionately benefit those with limited literacy;[35,36] however, only a very small proportion of patients with limited literacy have access to such programs.[28]

V. Theme 2—The Role of Information Technology in Health Literacy Research

There has been an explosion of creativity and investment in health information technologies. However, there is a significant risk that this current rapid expansion will worsen health disparities as many of the electronic systems will disproportionately benefit those with higher education and income.[37] The chief challenges are to ensure that people with limited literacy have access to technologies and that they are designed for ease of use by people with limited literacy. How will people get the technology? Will people be able to use technology?

A. Access to Technologies

While the internet has emerged as a major source of health information, access to and use of the internet to learn health information has been shown to be very strongly linked to health literacy.[25,38] However, this is a moving target and will need to be monitored as social norms regarding the internet evolve rapidly.[39] There is great potential for web-based projects and various authors have begun to explore how to deliver health information in a web-based fashion that is sensitive to literacy, culture, and linguistic needs.[40] We are on the cusp of a wide range of patient-facing technological advances in personal health records, smart phone-based health applications, and biometric monitoring systems, and yet a large percentage of community physicians work without even a rudimentary electronic health record. As such, the issue of access needs to be viewed from both the perspective of patient-facing technologies as well as basic electronic health record infrastructure.

B. User Interface

Sarkar and colleagues (in press, Journal of Health Communication) have shown that use of a patient portal system is linked to health literacy even when controlling for access. Attention is needed to simplify all aspects of the user interface with whatever form of technology that is being considered. Such simplification is clearly the goal of work led by Bickmore and colleagues who have explored the use of "embodied conversational agents"—animated computer characters—to interact with people (the character talks and the user responds with a touch-screen) in a variety of settings to promote health. Bickmore and colleagues (in press, Journal of Health Communication) have shown that people with limited health literacy and no computer literacy are able to and do use them, at least in a variety of study settings.

C. Behavioral Informatics

The chief focus of technology presentations at the HARC were oriented to behavioral informatics, i.e., information technologies (e.g., automated telephone calls, integrated electronic health record systems with patient portals, and computerized agents) that are designed to engage people in health activities. The value is clear; as health systems become automated, these tools allow for greater outreach, accountability, and standardization in the way health and healthcare is communicated to patients and families. Sarkar and colleagues compared the effectiveness of a diabetes self-management intervention using automated telephone calls with a nurse follow-up versus group medical visits and usual care.[41] Those receiving the automated calls reported better perceived diabetes care, communication, and both intervention arms documented improved self-care behaviors, fewer bed days, and less interference with daily activities. In a small pilot of an animated, computerized agent to standardize communication for an informed consent process, Bickmore et al. found patients to be more accepting of the technology even compared to human interactions, although no differences in knowledge acquisition were noted.[42] Both of these studies highlight the potential value of health technologies for engaging patients, particularly those with limited health literacy, yet more research is needed to better document the link between these interventions and health outcomes.

D. Electronic Health Records

A common and important focus of health information technology is electronic health records. Electronic health records, however, was not a significant focus of the HARC meeting. This is almost certainly due to the fact that this is completely assumed to be an uncontroversial necessity.

VI. Conference Agenda

Schedule of Events—Health Literacy Annual Research Conference 2009
National Academy of Sciences, Washington, DC

Time	Day 1: Monday October 19, 2009
8:00am–9:00am	Breakfast/Registration
9:00am–11:00am	NIH Gaps and Priorities Session, Moderator Ruth Parker
11:00am–12:00pm	Gaps/Priorities Small Group Breakout Sessions/ Box Lunch
12:00pm–12:45pm	Keynote Address: **David C. Baker, MD, MPH** Michael A. Gertz Professor in Medicine, Chief, Division of General Internal Medicine, Feinberg School of Medicine, Northwestern University
1:00pm–2:15pm	Abstract I—Oral Presentations, Moderator: Joanne Schwartzberg 1. Ian Bennett, University of Pennsylvania: "Trust of Physicians Mediates the Association of Literacy with Perceived Efficacy of Patient-Physician Interactions Among Mothers of Early Preterm Infants" 2. Ariella Herman, UCLA: "Empowering low-income parents to reduce excess pediatric emergency room and clinic visits through health literacy" 3. Stacy Bailey, Northwestern University: "Universal Medication Schedule to Improve Patient Understanding of Prescription Drug Instructions" 4. H Shonna Yin, New York University School of Medicine: "Parent Medication Administration Errors: Role of Dosing Instruments and Health Literacy"
2:30pm–3:45pm	Invited Panel A—Measurement, Moderator: Terry Davis Speakers: Elizabeth Hahn, Lauren McCormack, Russell Rothman
4:00pm–5:15pm	Invited Panel B—Health Literacy and Verbal Interactions, Moderator: Scott Ratzan Speakers: Kathy Mazur, Don Rubin, Debra Roter
5:30pm–7:00pm	Reception/Poster Session *For Directions to hotel, see map in your blue registration folder*

Time	Day 2: Tuesday October 20, 2009
8:00am–8:30am	Breakfast
8:30am–9:45am	Abstract II—Oral Presentations, Moderator: Irene Dankwa-Mullan 1. Drenna Waldrop-Valverde, University of Miami Miller School of Medicine: "Health Literacy and Prospective Memory in HIV Seropositive Individuals" 2. Rebecca Sudore, UCSF: "Uncertainty of Advance Care Planning Treatment Preferences Among Diverse Older Adults" 3. Raymond Ownby, Nova Southeastern University: "Health Literacy is Related to Problem Solving Skills" 4. Susan J. Shaw, University of Arizona: "Measuring Health Literacy Across Diverse Populations"
10:00am–10:45am	Keynote Address—**Anne Beal, MD, MPH**, President, Aetna Foundation
10:45am:	*Presentation of Sabra Woolley Memorial Award for highest rated abstract—Linda Harris*
11:00am–12:15pm	Invited Panel C—Health Information Technology Interventions, Moderator: Michael Paasche-Orlow Speakers: Timothy Bickmore, Dean Schillinger, Mike Wolf
11:00am–12:15pm	Invited Panel D—Organizational Assessment and Change, Moderator: Rima Rudd Speakers: Julie Gazmararian, Matthew Wynia, Beverly Weidmer
12:30pm–2:00pm	1-on-1 Meetings with NIH Project Officers and/or Research Mentors and Box Lunch
12:30pm–2:00pm	Poster Session
2:00pm–3:15pm	Abstract III—Oral Presentations, Moderator: Cindy Brach 1. Sian Smith, University of Sydney: "Supporting informed choices about bowel cancer screening among adults with lower levels of education and literacy: A randomized controlled trail of a decision aid" 2. Kerri L. Cavanaugh, Vanderbilt University Medical Center: "Low diabetes numeracy predicts worse glycemic control"

	3. Oana Grone, HPH Catalonian network: "Results of an evaluation of the health literacy environment in Catalan hospitals"
	4. Boyd H. Davis, University of North Carolina-Charlotte: "Vignettes and photovellas to enhance training for workers with limited English"
3:30pm–4:00pm	Final Session/Evaluations *If you are unable to complete your evaluation at the conference, be sure to visit our website and complete it online: http://www.bumc.bu.edu/healthliteracyconference/*

Reference List

1. National Institutes of Health Program Announcement: Understanding and Promoting Health Literacy. http://grants.nih.gov/grants/guide/pa-files/PAR-07-020.html. 2007.
2. Nielsen-Bohlman LT, Panzer AM, Hamlin B, Kindig DA. Institute of Medicine. Health Literacy: A Prescription to End Confusion. Committee on Health Literacy, Board on Neuroscience and Behavioral Health. 2004. Washington DC, National Academies Press.
3. Paasche-Orlow MK, Schillinger D, Greene SM, Wagner EH. How health care systems can begin to address the challenge of limited literacy. *J Gen Intern Med* 2006; 21(8):884-887.
4. Paasche-Orlow MK, Wolf MS. The causal pathways linking health literacy to health outcomes. *Am J Health Behav* 2007; 31 Suppl 1:S19-S26.
5. National Assessment of Adult Literacy (NAAL) http://nces.ed.gov/naal/kf_demographics.asp
6. Kutner, M., Greenberg, E., Jin,Y., and Paulsen, C. (2006). *The Health Literacy of America's Adults: Results From the 2003 National Assessment of Adult Literacy* (NCES 2006–483).U.S.Department of Education.Washington, DC: National Center for Education Statistics.
7. Paasche-Orlow MK, Parker RM, Gazmararian JA, Nielsen-Bohlman LT, Rudd RR. The prevalence of limited health literacy. *J Gen Intern Med* 2005; 20(2):175-184.
8. Volandes AE, Paasche-Orlow M, Gillick MR, Cook EF, Shaykevich S, Abbo ED, et al. Health Literacy not Race Predicts End-of-Life Care Preferences. *J Palliat Med* 2008; 11(5):754-762.
9. Osborn CY, Paasche-Orlow MK, Davis TC, Wolf MS. Health literacy: an overlooked factor in understanding HIV health disparities. Am J Prev Med. 2007 Nov;33(5):374-8.
10. Kalichman SC, Ramachandran B, Catz S. Adherence to combination antiretroviral therapies in HIV patients of low health literacy. *J Gen Intern Med* 1999; 14(5):267-273.
11. Wilson FL, Racine E, Tekieli V, Williams B. Literacy, readability and cultural barriers: critical factors to consider when educating older African Americans about anticoagulation therapy. *J Clin Nurs* 2003; 12(2):275-282.
12. Kalichman SC, Rompa D. Functional health literacy is associated with health status and health-related knowledge in people living with HIV-AIDS. *J Acquir Immune Defic Syndr* 2000; 25(4):337-344.

13. Sudore RL, Mehta KM, Simonsick EM, Harris TB, Newman AB, Satterfield S et al. Limited literacy in older people and disparities in health and healthcare access. *J Am Geriatr Soc* 2006; 54(5):770-776.
14. Sentell TL, Halpin HA. Importance of adult literacy in understanding health disparities. *J Gen Intern Med* 2006; 21(8):862-866.
15. Saha S. Improving literacy as a means to reducing health disparities. *J Gen Intern Med* 2006; 21(8):893-895.
16. Rothman RL, DeWalt DA, Malone R, Bryant B, Shintani A, Crigler B et al. Influence of patient literacy on the effectiveness of a primary care-based diabetes disease management program. *JAMA* 2004; 292(14):1711-1716.
17. Howard DH, Sentell T, Gazmararian JA. Impact of health literacy on socioeconomic and racial differences in health in an elderly population. *J Gen Intern Med* 2006; 21(8):857-861.
18. Lindau ST, Basu A, Leitsch SA. Health literacy as a predictor of follow-up after an abnormal Pap smear: a prospective study. *J Gen Intern Med* 2006; 21(8):829-834.
19. Volandes AE, Paasche-Orlow MK. Health literacy, health inequality and a just healthcare system. *Am J Bioeth* 2007; 7(11):5-10.
20. National Institutes of Health Program Announcement: Understanding and Promoting Health Literacy. http://grants.nih.gov/grants/guide/pa-files/PAR-07-020.html. 2007.
21. Berkman ND, Dewalt DA, Pignone MP, Sheridan SL, Lohr KN, Lux L, Sutton SF, Swinson T, Bonito AJ. Literacy and health outcomes. Evid Rep Technol Assess (Summ). 2004 Jan;(87):1-8. Review.
22. Ad Hoc Committee on Health Literacy, American Medical Association Council on Scientific Affairs. Health literacy: report of the Council on Scientific Affairs. JAMA. 1999;281:552–7.
23. Joint Commission for the Accreditation of Hospital Organization (JCAHO). What Did the Doctor Say? Improving Health Literacy to Protect Patient Safety. Health Care at the Crossroads Report. Oakbrook, IL, 2007. February.
24. Kutner, M., Greenberg, E., Jin,Y., Boyle, B.,Hsu,Y., and Dunleavy, E. (2007). Literacy in Everyday Life: Results From the 2003 National Assessment of Adult Literacy (NCES 2007–480).U.S.Department of Education. Washington, DC National Center for Education Statistics.
25. Kutner, M., Greenberg, E., Jin,Y., and Paulsen, C (2006). The Health Literacy of America's Adults: Results From the 2003 National Assessment of Adult Literacy (NCES 2006–483). Washington, DC, U.S.Department of Education: National Center for Education Statistics.
26. Osborn CY, P.-O. M., Davis TC, Wolf MS. (2007). "Health literacy: an overlooked factor in understanding HIV health disparities." Am J Prev Med **33**(5): 374-8.
27. Volandes AE, P.-O. M., Gillick MR, Cook EF, Shaykevich S, Abbo ED, Lehmann L. (2008). "Health literacy not race predicts end-of-life care preferences." J Palliat Med **11**(5): 754-62.
28. Paasche-Orlow, M. K., Schillinger, Dean, Greene, Sarah M, and Wagner, Edward H (2006). "How Health Care Systems Can Begin to Address the Challenge of Limited Literacy " J Gen Intern Med **21**(8): 884-887.
29. Davidoff AJ, S. B., Shaffer T, Shoemaker JS, Kim M, Zacker C (2010). "Lessons Learned: Who Didn't Enroll In Medicare Drug Coverage In 2006, And Why?" Health Aff (Millwood).
30. Ettner SL, S. N., Duru OK, Turk N, Quiter E, Schmittdiel J, Mangione CM (2010). "Entering and exiting the medicare part d coverage gap: role of comorbidities and demographics." J Gen Intern Med **25**(6): 568-74.
31. Castro CM, W. C., Wang F, Schillinger D (2007). "Babel babble: physicians' use of unclarified medical jargon with patients." Am J Health Behav **31**(Suppl 1): S85-95.

32. Schillinger D, P. J., Grumbach K, Wang F, Wilson C, Daher C, Leong-Grotz K, Castro C, Bindman AB (2003). "Closing the loop: physician communication with diabetic patients who have low health literacy." Arch Intern Med **163**(1): 83-90.
33. Fang MC, P. P., Machtinger EL, Schillinger D. (2009). "Language, literacy, and characterization of stroke among patients taking warfarin for stroke prevention: Implications for health communication." Patient Educ Couns 75(3): 403-10.
34. Carter-Pokras O, B. S., Lie D, Braddock CH 3rd; National Consortium for Multicultural Education for Health Professionals (2010). "Surmounting the unique challenges in health disparities education: a multi-institution qualitative study." J Gen Intern Med 25(Suppl 2): S108-14.
35. Rothman R, Malone R, Bryant B, Horlen C, DeWalt D, Pignone M. The relationship between literacy and glycemic control in a diabetes disease-management program. Diabetes Educ. 2004 Mar-Apr;30(2):263-73.
36. DeWalt DA, Pignone M, Malone R, Rawls C, Kosnar MC, George G, Bryant B, Rothman RL, Angel B. Development and pilot testing of a disease management program for low literacy patients with heart failure. Patient Educ Couns. 2004 Oct;55(1):78-86.
37. Viswanath K., Kreuter, MW. *Health Disparities, Communication Inequalities and E-health: A Commentary*. American Journal of Preventive Medicine. 2007; 32 (5 Suppl): S131-3.
38. Czaja SJ, S. J., Nair SN (2008). "Usability of the Medicare health web site." JAMA **300**(7): 790-2.
39. Samal L, Yeh HC, Gary-Webb TL, Jackson CL, Brancati FL. Computer and internet use of urban african americans with type 2 diabetes in relation to glycemic control, emergency department use, diabetes-related knowledge, and health literacy. Diabetes Care. 2010 Jan;33(1):e9.
40. Neuhauser L, Kreps GL. Online cancer communication: meeting the literacy, cultural and linguistic needs of diverse audiences. Patient Educ Couns. 2008 Jun;71(3):365-77.
41. Sarkar U, H. M., Gupta R, Tang A, Murphy E, Seligman HK, Shojania KG, Schillinger D (2008). "Use of an interactive, telephone-based self-management support program to identify adverse events among ambulatory diabetes patients." J Gen Intern Med **23**(4): 459-65.
42. Bickmore TW, P. L., Paasche-Orlow MK (2009). "Using computer agents to explain medical documents to patients with low health literacy." Patient Educ Couns **75**(3): 315-20.